W. Distler · L. Beck (Eds.)

Endorphins
in Reproduction
and Stress

With 44 Figures

Springer-Verlag Berlin Heidelberg New York
London Paris Tokyo Hong Kong Barcelona

Professor Dr. med. WOLFGANG DISTLER

Professor Dr. med. LUTWIN BECK

Universitäts-Frauenklinik
Moorenstraße 5
4000 Düsseldorf, FRG

ISBN 3-540-52736-2 Springer-Verlag Berlin Heidelberg New York
ISBN 0-387-52736-2 Springer-Verlag New York Berlin Heidelberg

Library of Congress Cataloging-in-Publication Data. Endorphins in human reproduction and stress response / W. Distler, L. Beck (eds). p.cm. Papers from a workshop conference held in October 1989 at he Dept. of Obstetrics and Gynecology of the University of Düsseldorf. Includes index. ISBN 3-540-52736-2 (alk. paper). – – ISBN 0-387-52736-2 (alk. paper) 1. Endorphins – –Physiological effect – –Congresses. 2. Human reproduction – –Endocrine aspects – –Congresses. 3. Stress (Physiology) – –Congresses. 4. Neuroendocrinology – –Congresses. I. Distler, Wolfgang. II. Beck, Lutwin. [DNLM: 1. Endorphins – –physiology – –congresses. 2. Reproduction – –physiology – congresses. 3. Stress, Psychological – –physiopathology – –congresses. 4. Stress, Psychological – physiopathology – congresses. WQ 205 E567 1989] QP552.E53E53 1990 612.6 – –dc20 DNLM/DLC for Library of Congress.

© Springer-Verlag Berlin Heidelberg 1990
Printed in Germany

The use of registered names, trademarks, etc. in this publication does not imply, even in the absence of a specific statement, that such names are exempt from the relevant protective laws and regulations and therefore free for general use.

Product liability: The publisher can give no guarantee for information about drug dosage and application thereof contained in this book. In every individual case the respective user must check its accuracy by consulting other pharmaceutical literature.

Typesetting: Pure Tech Corporation, India
2121/3130-543210 – Printed on acid-free paper

Preface

The last frontier of knowledge does not lie in the center of the earth or on the surface of some distant planet. The last frontier is within us: it is the human brain.

The idea that neurons secrete peptides was first proposed by Scharrer and Scharrer (1940). Thereafter, the isolation and characterization of numerous brain peptides stimulated the discovery of their cellular receptors in the central nervous system. However, in the case of the opioid peptides, the opiate receptor recognition and the development of a specific bioassay came first and provided the means to isolate the opiate-like peptides.

Pert and Snyder (1973) were the first to recognize opiate receptors. A little later two endogenous ligands (leu-enkephalin and met-enkephalin) were identified (Hughes et al. 1975). It came as a surprise that the met-enkephalin amino acid sequence was identical to the residue 61-65 of β-lipotropin (β-LPH), which had been first described years ago by Li (1964). In addition, it became apparent that a number of peptide fragments originated from β-LPH. The fragment of β-LPH containing the amino acid residue sequence 61-76 was later named α-endorphin. Two other fragments, γ-endorphin and δ-endorphin, proved to be identical to β-LPH 61-77 and β-LPH 61-87, respectively. β-Endorphin (β-LPH 61-91) was independently isolated by Bradbury (1976) and showed the greatest opiate-like activity of all endorphins. In 1979 and 1980 further characterization of dynorphin, α-neoendorphin, and (H-) endorphin expended the number of endogenous ligands for the opiate receptors.

In recent years it has become increasingly apparent that endogenous opioids exert profound effects on the endocrine system. Therefore the topics of a workshop conference, held in October 1989 at the Department of Obstetrics and Gynecology of the University of Düsseldorf, were intended to cover relevant aspects of opioid neuroendocrinology. The contributions collected in this volume attempt to give an overview of the current state of knowledge regarding opioid peptide regulation of reproductive function and stress response.

With the collaboration of the Arbeitsgemeinschaft für gynäkologische Endokrinologie der Deutschen Gesellschaft für Gynäkologie und Geburtshilfe, the interest in the meeting was extremely encouraging, as were the reactions from participants after the conference. It is important to us to acknowledge the financial support given by the Deutsche Gesellschaft für Endokrinologie, Ferring Arzneimittel GmbH, Nourypharma GmbH, Bayer AG, Organon GmbH,

Cilag GmbH, and Schering AG.Further more, our sincere appreciation and gratitude are due to all the contributors, who prepared their manuscripts meticulously, and to Mrs. Sieglinde El-Bahay for her secretarial assistance. Since only a small number of speakers could be invited, rapid publication of this book was considered to be of crucial importance; the unusual speed of publication would not have been possible without the excellent work of Springer-Verlag.

Düsseldorf, Summer 1990   WOLFGANG DISTLER
                                                                LUTWIN BECK

References

Bradbury AF (1976) C fragment of lipotropin has a high affinity for brain opiate receptors. Nature 260:793

Hughes J, Smith TW, Kosterlitz HW, Fothergill LA, Morgan BA, Morris HR (1975) Identification of two related pentapeptides from the brain with potent opiate agonist activity. Nature 258:577-579

Li CH (1964) Lipotropin, a new active peptide from pituitary glands. Nature 201:924-925

Pert CB, Snyder SH (1973) Opiate receptor: Demonstration in nervous tissue. Science 201:924-925

Scharrer E, Scharrer B (1940) Secretory cells within the hypothalamus. Proc Assoc Res Nerv Ment Dis 20:170-194

Contents

List of Contributors

ALLOLIO, B., Medizinische Universitäts-Klinik II, Krankenhaus Merheim, Ostmerheimer Straße 200, 5000 Köln 91, FRG

ALMEIDA, O.F.X., Institut für Pharmakologie, Toxikologie und Pharmazie der Tierärztlichen Fakultät der Ludwig-Maximilian-Universität, Königinstraße 16, 8000 München 22, FRG

AMATO, F., Department of Obstetrics and Gynecology, University of Modena, Via del Pozzo 71, 41100 Modena, Italy

ANGIONI, S., Department of Obstetrics and Gynecology, University of Modena, Via del Pozza 71, 41100 Modena, Italy

BARTLETT, J.M.S., Institut für Reproduktionsmedizin der Westfälischen Wilhelms-Universität, Steinfurter Straße 107, 4400 Münster, FRG

BENSCH, J., Abteilung für Klinische und Experimentelle Endokrinologie, Universitäts-Frauenklinik Eppendorf, Martinistraße 52, 2000 Hamburg 20, FRG

BETTELLI, S., Department of Obstetrics and Gynecology, University of Modena, Via del Pozzo 71, 41100 Modena, Italy

BORN, J., Medizinische Klinik und Poliklinik der Universität, Robert-Koch-Straße 9, 7900 Ulm, FRG

BRAENDLE, W.L., Abteilung für Klinische und Experimentelle Endokrinologie, Universitäts-Frauenklinik Eppendorf, Martinistraße 52, 2000 Hamburg 20, FRG

COMITINI, G., Department of Obstetrics and Gynecology, University of Modena, Via del Pozzo 71, 41100 Modena, Italy

DEUSS, U., Medizinische Universitäts-Klinik II, Krankenhaus Merheim, Ostmerheimer Straße 200, 5000 Köln 91, FRG

DISTLER, W., Universitäts-Frauenklinik, Moorenstraße 5, 4000 Düsseldorf, FRG

FEHM, H.L., Medizinische Klinik und Poliklinik der Universität, Robert-Koch-Straße 9, 7900 Ulm, FRG

GALASSI, M.C., Department of Obstetrics and Gynecology, University of Modena, Via del Pozzo 71, 41100 Modena, Italy

GENAZZANI, A.R., Department of Obstetrics and Gynecology, University of Modena, Via del Pozzo 71, 41100 Modena, Italy

GROSSMAN, A., Department of Endocrinology, St. Bartholomew's Hospital, West Smithfield, London EC1A 7BE, England

HOHTARI, H., The Finninsh Foundation of Exercise and Sports Medicine, 00290 Helsinki, Finland

JARRY, H., Universitäts-Frauenklinik, Abteilung für Klinische und Experimentelle Endokrinologie, Robert-Koch-Straße 40, 3400 Göttingen, FRG

KOCH, G., Rudolf-Buchheim-Institut für Pharmakologie, Universität Gießen, Frankfurter Straße 107, 6300 Gießen, FRG

KRAMER, D., Rudolf-Buchheim-Institut für Pharmakologie, Universität Gießen, Frankfurter Straße 107, 6300 Gießen, FRG

LAATIKAINEN, T., Departments of Obstetrics and Gynecology, Helsinki University Central Hospital, Haartmaninkatu 2, 00290 Helsinki, Finland

LEONHARDT, S., Universitäts-Frauenklinik, Abteilung für Klinische und Experimentelle Endokrinologie, Robert-Koch-Straße 40, 3400 Göttingen, FRG

PETRAGLIA, F., Department of Obstetrics and Gynecology, University of Modena, Via del Pozzo 71, 41100 Modena, Italy

PFEIFFER, A., Medizinische Klinik und Poliklinik, Universität Bochum, Gilsingerstraße 14, 4630 Bochum, FRG

PFEIFFER, D.G., Universitäts-Frauenklinik Großhadern, Marchionini 15, 8000 München 70, FRG

PRETI, B., Department of Obstetrics and Gynecology, University of Modena, Via del Pozzo 71, 41100 Modena, Italy

RAHKILA, P., Research Unit for Sports and Physical Fitness, Jyväskylä, Finland

REINCKE, M., Medizinische Universitäts-Klinik II, Krankenhaus Merheim, Ostmerheimer Straße 200, 5000 Köln 91, FRG

SCHULTE, H.M., Medizinische Klinik, Universität Kiel, Schittenhelmstraße 12, 2300 Kiel, FRG

SWEEP, C.G.J., Rudolf Magnus Institute, Department for Pharmacology, University of Utrecht, Vondellaan 6, 3521 GD Utrecht, The Netherlands

SZALAY, K.SZ., Institute of Experimental Medicine, Hungarian Academy of Sciences, POB 67, 1450 Budapest, Hungary

TESCHEMACHER, H., Rudolf-Buchheim-Institut für Pharmakologie, Universität Gießen, Frankfurter Straße 107, 6300 Gießen, FRG

TESORIO, N., Department of Obstetrics and Gynecology, University of Modena, Via del Pozzo 71, 41100 Modena, Italy

TORRES NORIEGA, J., Universitäts-Frauenklinik, Abteilung für Klinische und Experimentelle Endokrinologie, Robert-Koch-Straße 40, 3400 Göttingen, FRG

WESTHOF, G., Abteilung für Klinische und Experimentelle Endokrinologie, Universitäts-Frauenklinik Eppendorf, Martinistraße 52, 2000 Hamburg 20, FRG

WIEDEMANN, K., Rudolf-Buchheim-Institut für Pharmakologie, Universität Gießen, Frankfurter Straße 107, 6300 Gießen, FRG

WIEGANT, V.M., Rudolf Magnus Institute, Department for Pharmacology, University of Utrecht, Vondellaan 6, 3521 GD Utrecht, The Netherlands

WINKELMANN, W., Medizinsiche Universitäts-Klinik II, Krankenhaus Merheim, Ostmerheimer Straße 200, 5000 Köln 91, FRG

WUTTKE, W., Universitäts-Frauenklinik, Abteilung für Klinische und Experimentelle Endokrinologie, Robert-Koch-Straße 40, 3400 Göttingen, FRG

Opioids and Endocrine Secretion

Opioid Control of Gonadotropin Secretion

A.R. Genazzani, F. Petraglia, S. Angioni, G. Comitini, S. Bettelli, B. Preti, f. Amato, N. Tesorio, and M.C. Galassi

Introduction

Among the various neuropeptides which regulate gonadotropin secretion, endogenous opioid peptides (EOP) play an important role. Substantial evidence suggests a possible key function of for these peptides in the control of female reproduction. Infertility, for example, is typical in members of both sexes who abuse opiates. The major target of EOP in regulating reproductive function is control of the secretion of luteinizing hormone (LH), inhibiting the activity of hypothalamic neurons which produce gonadotropin-releasing hormone (GnRH). A possible action of opioids on pituitary and/or gonadal hormone secretion has also been demonstrated.

The existence of three families of endogenous opioid peptide and their wide distribution in brain and in peripheral tissues prompts the question of which is most involved in the control of reproductive function.

The various endogenous opioid peptides are derived from three different precursors: proopiomelanocortin (POMC), preproenkephalin A and preproenkephalin B. The carboxyl end of POMC with its terminal 31 aa constitutes β-endorphin (β-End), one of the main EOPs. Other POMC-related peptides without opioid activity are β-lipotropin and adrenocorticotropic hormone (ACTH). Methionine-enkephalin (M-E) derives, from the proteolytic processing of preproenkephalin A, while the major product of preproenkephalin B is dynorphin (Dyn) (Facchinetti et al. 1987). A further differentiation among the three opioid peptide families is the selective binding to specific opioid receptors. At least five are now recognized: μ, κ, δ, σ, and ε (Paterson et al. 1983). β-End seems to work on μ– and ε-receptors, Dyn on κ-receptors, and M-E on δ-receptors. Of the defined receptor agonists and antagonists, naloxone is the most-used antagonist. It is not selective; at low doses it is effective on μ-receptors, while at higher doses it also blocks κ– and σ–receptors.

The highest concentration of β–End is in the mediobasal hypothalamus, particularly in the arcuate nuclei and the median eminence. M-E is probably the most widely distributed EOP in the brain; the highest concentrations are present in the globus pallidus and substantia nigra. The hypothalamus is the area of the brain in which the neurons producing Dyn are mostly localized (Watson et al. 1982).

Studies in Rats

Experimental studies have clarified (a) which of the EOPs is most involved in the control of LH secretion, (b) the target of EOPs, and (c) their mechanism of action. Injection of β-End, M-E, and Dyn into rat brain decreases plasma LH levels. To determine the EOP and/or the specific opiate receptor subtype involved in the regulation of LH secretion, antisera directed at the different EOPs or receptor antagonists were administered in rats. Administration of anti-β-End serum both centrally and peripherally caused a significant rise in plasma LH levels. Antiserum against Dyn had less effect, while anti-M–E had no effect (Schultz et al. 1981; Forman et al. 1983). These data agree with the evidence that naloxone is more potent than other κ or δ-receptor specific antagonists in increasing LH levels in various experimental models (Panerai et al. 1985). β-End is therefore the endogenous ligand with the preeminent role in inhibiting LH secretion.

Multiple studies have shown that EOP modulates LH secretion, acting in the central nervous system. A naloxone-induced rise in serum LH levels may be blocked by GnRH antagonists, which supports the hypothesis that GnRH is a target of EOP action (Blank and Roberts 1982). Furthermore, naloxone stimulates GnRH from hypothalamus explants and increases GnRH levels in the hypophyseal portal circulation (Ramunssen et al. 1983; Sarkar and Yen 1985). Moreover, excluding a pituitary site of action, EOPs do not modify basal or GnRH-induced LH release from pituitary cells in vitro and do not influence the secretory response to GnRH in vivo (Cicero et al. 1979). On the contrary, a direct effect of β-End on pituitary LH secretion in vitro has also been reported (Blank et al. 1986). On the basis of this last observation, a putative role of β-End circulating in the systemic bloodstream has been suggested. However, plasma β-End does not seem to have an important part in the regulatory effect of EOP on gonadotropin secretion; changes in plasma β-End concentration are not followed by inverse changes in plasma LH levels (Petraglia et al. 1988b). It can therefore be ruled out that peripheral β-End has a major role to play.

Within the hypothalamus, EOP inhibits the activity of GnRH-producing neurons both directly and via modulation of neurotransmitter afferences. Inhibition of the stimulatory noradrenergic signals or/and increase of inhibitory serotoninergic or dopaminergic influences have been shown to occur in the mechanism of LH inhibition by EOP (Kalra and Kalra 1983).

The action of EOP on the hypothalamus-pituitary-ovarian (HPO) axis is influenced by gonadal steroids. The LH response to naloxone changes during the estrous cycle in female rats suggests that phyisiological changes in gonadal steroids modify the activity of EOP. On the day of proestrus, at the time of highest plasma LH levels, naloxone does not further stimulate LH secretion. Administration of pharmacological doses of estradiol benzoate to adult female rats is also followed by the disappearance of rise in LH due to naloxone (Petraglia et al. 1986b). Moreover, naloxone and opiate agonists do not change

LH levels in castrated rats, suggesting that inadequate gonadal steroid levels may reduce the influence of opioids on LH release (Bhanot and Wilkinson 1983), and, indeed, replacement therapy with gonadal steroids restores normal responsiveness to opiate antagonists (Petraglia et al. 1984). On the basis of these results, a role of EOP in the transmission of gonadal feedback signals to the brain structures has been hypothesized (Yen 1984).

An important role of EOP in stress-induced hypogonadotropinemia was also shown. Both naloxone and antisera raised against β-End or Dyn reversed the stress-induced decrease of plasma LH (Petraglia et al. 1986d).

Studies in Humans

In humans, naloxone administration stimulates LH secretion with an age-related difference. Naloxone administered to prepubertal children does not significantly change plasma LH levels (Fraioli et al. 1984; Mauras et al. 1986). It is well known that in the prepubertal period there is no pulsatile LH secretion, with plasma follicle-stimulating hormone levels higher than LH. During pubertal maturation this secretory pattern undergoes important changes. It is hypothesized that these changes are related to the disappareance of an inhibiting factor or to the development of a stimulatory pathway. The hypothesis of a gonadostat seems to be the most plausible. It has been suggested that EOP has the role of gonadostat. Plasma LH levels rise following naloxone administration in children of both sexes at advanced stages of pubertal maturation (Petraglia et al. 1986a). In children with gonadal dysgenesis or delayed puberty, naloxone causes no rise in plasma LH levels (Petraglia et al. 1986a, 1988a). Therefore, it has been suggested that the activity of EOP on LH reflects the maturation of the hypothalamus-pituitary-gonadal axis.

Changes of opioid control of LH secretion during the menstrual cycle are also described: the effect of naloxone is evident during the luteal phase but not during follicular phase (Quigley and Yen 1980; Snowden et al. 1984). The stimulatory activity of naloxone on LH is present from the preovulatory days. The naloxone-induced rise in LH is related to the circulating estradiol levels. The opioid pathway is most probably very important in the hypothalamic control of the ovulatory mechanisms. The changes of opioid activity during the menstrual cycle are not evident using opiate agonists. Morphine injection inhibits plasma LH levels in all patients, irrespective of phase in the menstrual cycle (Petraglia et al. 1986c). The response to injected naloxone is absent in patients with hypothalamic amenorrhea (Petraglia et al. 1985b); following GnRH pulsatile or gonadotropin therapies, a normal LH response to naloxone is restored (Nappi et al. 1987). It is interesting that in patients taking hormonal contraceptives, the blocking of ovulation inhibits the LH response to naloxone, despite the presence of steroid hormones (Casper et al. 1984). By contrast, hyperprolactinemic patients or patients with polycystic ovary disease, despite low plasma levels of gonadal steroids, show a significant rise in plasma LH

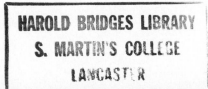

following naloxone injection (Petraglia et al. 1987; Cumming et al. 1984; Grossman et al. 1980).

During the postmenopausal period opioid action on LH secretion changes again: after physiological or surgical menopause naloxone does not increase plasma LH levels (Petraglia et al. 1985a). Injection of β-End or demorphine also fails to reduce LH plasma levels in postmenopausal women (Petraglia et al. 1985c; Reid et al. 1983). Replacement therapy with steroids restores EOP action in modulating gonadotropin secretion (Shoupe et al. 1985). Treatment with dopamine agonists also restores the responce of LH to naloxone (Melis et al. 1981).

Conclusion

These studies indicate that opioid peptides regulate gonadotropin secretion, action on hypothalamic GnRH. This effect results from the interaction with gonadal steroid and neurotransmitter activities. The inhibitory effect of opioids on circulating LH represents one of the key factors modulating the activity of the hypothalamus-pituitary-ovarian axis.

References

Bhanot R, Wilkinson M (1983) Opiatergic control of LH secretion is eliminated by gonadectomy. Endocrinology 112:399-401
Blank MS, Roberts DL (1982) Antagonist of gonadotropin-releasing hormone blocks naloxone-induced elevations in serum luteinizing hormone. Neuroendocrinology 35:308-312
Blank MS, Fabbria A, Catt KJ, Dufau ML (1986) Inhibition of luteinizing hormone release by morphine and endogenous opiates in cultured pituitary cells. Endocrinology 118:2097-2101
Casper RF, Bhanot R, Wilkinson M (1984) Prolonged elevation of hypothalamic opioid peptide activity in women taking oral contraceptives. J Clin Endocrinol Metab 58:582-584
Cicero TJ, Schainker BA, Meyer ER (1979) Endogenous opioids participate in the regulation of the hypothalamic-pituitary- luteinizing hormone axis and testosterone negative feedback control of luteinizing hormone. Endocrinology 104:1286-1289
Cumming DC, Reid RL, Quigley ME, Rebar RW, Yen SSC (1984) Evidence for decreased endogenous dopamine and opioid inhibitory influences on LH secretion in polycystic ovary syndrome. Clin Endocrinol (Oxf) 20:643-647
Facchinetti F, Petraglia F, Genazzani AR (1987) Localization and expression of the three opioid systems. Semin Reprod Endocrinol 5:103-113
Forman LJ, Sonntag WE, Meites J (1983) Elevation of plasma LH in response to systemic injection of β-endorphin antiserum in adult male rats. Proc Soc Exp Biol Med 173: 14-17
Fraioli F, Cappa M, Fabbri A, Gnessi L, Moretti C, Borelli P, Isidori A (1984) Lack of endogenous inhibitory tone on LH secretion in early puberty. Clin Endocrinol (Oxf) 20: 299-303
Grossman A, Moult PJ, McIntyre H, Evans J, Silverstone T, Rees LH, Bessner MG (1980) Opiate mediation of amenorrhea in hyperprolactinemia and weight-loss related amenorrhea. Clin Endocrinol (Oxf) 17: 379-383

Kalra SP, Kalra PS (1983) Neural regulation of luteinizing hormone secretion in the rat. Endocr Rev 4: 311-351

Mauras N, Veidhuis JD, Rogol L (1986) Role of endogenous opioid in pubertal maturation: opposing action of naltrexone in prepubertal and late pubertal boys. J Clin Endocrinol Metab 63: 1256-1260

Melis GB, Cagnacci A, Gambacciani M, Paoletti AM, Caffi T, Fioretti P (1981) Chronic bromocriptine administration restores luteinizing hormone response to naloxone in postmenopausal women. Neuroendocrinology 47: 159-163

Nappi C, Petraglia F, di Meo G, Minutolo M, Genazzani AR, Montemagno U (1987) Opioid regulation of LH secretion in amenorrheic patients following therapies of induction of ovulation. Fertil Steril 47: 579-582

Panerai AE, Petraglia F, Sacerdote P, Genazzani AR (1985) Mainly μ-opiate receptors are involved in luteinizing hormone and prolactin secretion. Endocrinology 117: 1096-1099

Paterson SJ, Robson LE, Kosterlitz HW (1983) Classification of opiate receptors. Br Med Bull 39: 31-40

Petraglia F, Locatelli V, Penalva A, Cocchi D, Genazzani AR, Muller EE (1984) Gonadal steroids modulation of naloxone-induced LH secretion in the rat. J Endocrinol 101: 33-39

Petraglia F, Comitini G, d'Ambrogio G, Volpe A, Facchinetti F, Alessandrini G, Genazzani AR (1985a) Short term control effect of ovariectomy: the opioid control of LH secretion in fertile, climateric and postmenopausal women. J Clin Endocrinol Metab 8: 325-329

Petraglia F, d'Ambrogio G, Comitini G, Facchinetti F, Volpe A, Genazzani AR (1985b) Impairment of opioid control of luteinizing hormone secretion in mestrual disorders. Fertil Steril 43: 535- 540

Petraglia F, Degli-Ubereti EC, Transfortini G, Facchinetti F, Margutti A, Volpe A, Salvatori S, Tomatis R, Genazzani AR (1985c) Demorphin decreases plasma LH levels in human: evidence for a modulatory role of gonadal steroids. Peptides 8: 869-872

Petraglia F, Bernasconi S, Iughetti L, Loche S, Romanini F, Facchinetti F, Marcellini C, Genazzani AR (1986a) Naloxone- induced luteinizing hormone secretion in normal precocious and delayed puberty. J Clin Endocrinol Metab 63: 1112-1116

Petraglia F, Locatelli V, Facchinetti F, Bergamaschi M, Genazzani AR, Cocchi D (1986b) Oestrus cycle-related LH responsiveness to naloxone: effect of high oestrogen levels on the activity of opioid receptors. J Endocrinol 108: 89-94

Petraglia F, Porro C, Facchinetti F, Cicoli C, Bertellini E, Volpe A, Barbieri GC, Genazzani AR (1986c) Opioid control of LH secretion in humans: menstrual cycle, menopause and aging reduce effect of naloxone but not of morphine. Life Sci 38: 2103-2110

Petraglia F, Vale W, Rivier C (1986d) Opioids act centrally to modulate stress-induced decrease of LH secretion in the rat. Endocrinology 112: 2209-2213

Petraglia F, de Leo V, Nappi C, Facchinetti F, Montemagno U, Brambilla F, Genazzani AR (1987) Differences in the opioid control of luteinizing hormone secretion between pathological and iatrogenic hyperprolactinemic states. J Clin Endocrinol Metab 64: 508-512

Petraglia F, Larizza D, Maghine M, Facchinetti F, Volpe A, Bernasconi S, Genazzani AR, Severi F (1988a) Impairment of the opioidergic control of luteinizing hormone secretion in Turner's syndrome: lack of effect of the gonadal steroid therapy. J Clin Endocrinol Metab 66: 1024-1028

Petraglia F, Panerai AE, Rivier C, Cocchi D, Genazzani AR (1988b) Opioid control of gonadotropin secretion. In: Genazzani AR, Montemagno U, Nappi C, Petraglia F (eds) The brain and female reproductive function. Parthenon Publ. Castherton, p 65

Quigley ME, Yen SSC (1980) The role of endogenous opiates on LH secretion during the menstrual cycle. J Clin Endocrinol Metab 51: 179-181

Ramunssen DD, Lui JH, Wolf PL, Yen SSC (1983) Endogenous opioid regulation of gonadotropin-releasing hormone release from human fetal hypothalamus in vitro. J Clin Endocrinol Metab 57: 881-884

Reid RL, Quigley ME, Yen SSC (1983) The disappearance of opioid regulation of gonadotropin secretion in post-menopausal women. J Clin Endocrinol Metab 57: 1107-1110

Sarkar DK, Yen SSC (1985) Hyperprolactinemia decreases luteinizing hormone-releasing hormone concentration in pituitary portal plasma: a possible role for β-endorphin as a mediator. Endocrinology 116: 2080-2085

Schultz R, Whilhelm A, Pirke KM, Gramsch G, Herz A (1981) β- Endorphin and dynorphin control serum LH level in immature female rats. Nature 294: 757-759

Shoupe D, Montz JF, Lobo AR (1985) The effects of estrogens and progestins on endogenous opioid activity in oophorectomized women. J Clin Endocrinol Metab 60: 178-181

Snowden UE, Khan-Dawood SF, Dawood MY (1984) The effect of naloxone on endogenous opioid regulation of pituitary gonadotropins and prolactin during the menstrual cycle. J Clin Endocrinol Metab 59: 292-296

Watson SJ, Khachaturian H, Akil H, Coy D, Goldstein A (1982) Comparison of the distribution of dynorphin system and enkephalin system in brain. Science 218: 1134-1137

Yen SSC (1984) Opiates and reproduction: studies in women. In: Delitala G (ed) Opioid modulation of endocrine function. Raven, New York, p 191

Neurochemical Regulation of the LHRH Pulse Generator

W. Wuttke, H. Jarry, S. Leonhardt, and J.Torres Noriega

Pituitary luteinizing hormone (LH) release occurs in episodes at more or less regular intervals. These episodes are subject to pulse and frequency modulation. Their basic features are particularly clearly revealed in gonadectomized individuals (Fig. 1). Changes in LH pulse amplitudes and frequencies during the

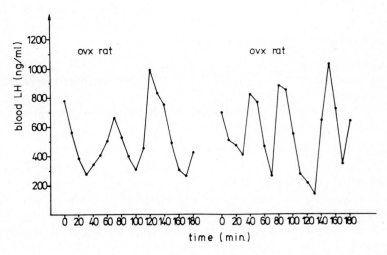

Fig. 1. Pulsatile LH pattern in two individual ovariectomized rats. The abrupt increases in blood LH levels are suggestive that a large number, if not all, of GnRH neurons activate phasically at the same time (phasic and synchronous activation). Only a GnRH release pattern like this is an appropriate signal for the pituitary to release LH episodes

estrous cycle of the rat have been described (Fox and Smith 1985). In ovariectomized or postmenopausal women the pulse frequency is approximately one pulse every 90 min, which corresponds to the frequency observed in steroid-intact, i.e., premenopausal women during the follicular phase. Here, however, the pulse amplitude is markedly reduced, due to a direct effect of circulating estrogens on the pituitary gonadotrophs (Cooper et al. 1973; for review see Crowley et al. 1985). From findings in the monkey (Knobil 1980) and in women it was concluded that in primates the hypothalamus plays only a permissive role, in that it releases gonadotropin releasing hormone (GnRH) prior to each LH episode in a rather stereotypic fashion, and it was indeed shown that administration of the same amount of GnRH at 90-min intervals through infusion pumps into hypothalamic amenorrheal women can restore normal ovulatory cycles (Leyendecker and Wildt 1983). Basically the same mechanisms operate in the rat hypothalamo-pituitary unit. In the rat the GnRH cells are not clustered in well-defined areas of the hypothalamus but are scattered in the anterior mediobasal hypothalamus, the preoptic area, and even into extrahypothalamic sites, such as the diagonal band of Broca and the medioseptal regions. In order for the hypothalamus to produce an appropriate signal for the pituitary, namely a GnRH pulse, the GnRH neurons have to increase their electrical activity synchronously. That this is indeed the case has been shown in the Rhesus monkey, in which multiunit activity in circumscribed areas of the mediobasal hypothalamus increased prior to the occurrence of LH pulses (Kaufman et al. 1985).

What drives the GnRH neurons?

At this point it should be emphasized again that a sharp   increase in GnRH release requires *simultaneous phasic* activation of GnRH neurons. Theoretically, several possibilities exist to explain such features:

1. A master oscillator drives GnRH neurons.
2. GnRH neurons form a self-organizing circuit which functions independently of other neuronal mechanisms.
3. Phasic activation and synchronization of GnRH neurons is brought about by two separate mechanisms.

There exists more or less scanty evidence for all three possibilities.

Possibility 1. A master oscillator was suggested by Rasmussen (1986), who tried to correlate LH pulsatility with brain stem activation. The reasoning behind this theoretical approach was that in phase and slightly out of phase synchronized CNS events can be explained by periodically occurring activation of the brain stem. Such periodic activation is obvious during sleep cycles. Rapid eye movement (REM) sleep phases occur approximately every 90 min. The author suggests that such cycles also occur during day time, of course without accompanying REM sleep phases, and that this drives the GnRH neurons. This approach could indeed explain why LH release during the night occurs in association with cyclic changes in sleep phases. There is, however, no experimental evidence for this hypothesis.

Possibility 2. From hypothalamic explants kept in short- term culture conditions in vitro, it is known that GnRH release occurs also in a pulsatile fashion (Bourguignon et al. 1989 a,b). Since these fragments were mostly taken from rat hypothalamus, they contain few, if any, GnRH perikarya. Hence, the release of axon terminals of these neurons is no longer governed by activity generated in the neurons. Nevertheless, there appears to be some degree of an axo-axonal interaction at the level of the median eminence which causes episodic release of GnRH. This would not in the true sense be a self-organizing circuit. The best evidence supporting the existence of a circuit of this kind stems from isolated cultivated GnRH neurons forming a diffuse network (Melrose et al. 1987). These GnRH cell cultures release their secretory product, namely GnRH, in a pulsatile fashion also, indicating that the neurons form a self- organizing circuit. Axosomatic synapses between GnRH neurons have also been demonstrated in intact hypothalami of juvenile monkeys (Thind and Goldsmith 1988), which indicates the possibility that a self organization resulting in pulsatile GnRH release may also function in vivo.

Possibility 3. There is increasing evidence that phasic neuronal activity can be induced by catecholamines. Particularly α_1-adrenoreceptive mechanisms are involved in phasic activation of a number of hypothalamic neurons, possibly including GnRH neurons (Kaufman et al. 1985). Stimulation of noradrenergic projection into the preoptic area excited the majority of neurons located there. Blockade of α_1-adrenoreceptors causes cessation of pulsatile LH release in ovariectomized rats. We demonstrated recently that this happens in the preoptic/anterior hypothalamic area and not in the mediobasal hypothalamus (Jarry et al. 1990a). This makes it likely that norepinephrine stimulates GnRH neurons directly. The magnocellular vasopressin neurons fire phasically upon appropriate osmotic stimulation, and it was shown electrophysiologically that phasic activation of these neurons can be prevented by blockade of α_1-receptors (Day et al. 1985). In an in vitro slice preparation of guinea pig hypothalamus, Condon et al. (1989) demonstrated that the α_1-agonist methoxamine induced phasic activation at irregular intervals for an extended period when present for a relatively short time. Hence, it seems very likely that norepinephrine is necessary for induction of phasic activation of hypothalamic neurons, and thus would appear also to be responsible for phasic activation of GnRH neurons. This norepinephrine-induced phasic activity, however, appears not to be synchronized. Thus, each GnRH neuron would release minibursts of GnRH, which would result in a continuous slight increase of GnRH in the portal vessels. This is obviously not the appropriate signal for the pituitary. Hence, we have to ask ourselves what mechanism might be responsible for synchronizing the norepinephrine-mediated phasic activation of GnRH neurons. We have good evidence that the ultimate synchronizing signal is a GABAergic mechanism (Jarry et al. 1988). The rates of release of GABA (γ-aminobutyric acid) in the preoptic/anterior hypothalamic area (the structure with the most GnRH neurons) in ovariectomized rats are high at times when LH levels are either decreasing or low. Only prior to the occurrence of LH episodes were preoptic GABA release rates drastically reduced. It thus appears that the GnRH neurons are subject to a tonic inhibitory effect of GABA, which is relieved simultaneously resulting in synchronous activation of GnRH neurons. The reason for the simultaneous relief of GABAergic inhibition remains obscure at present. The integrated interplay between a noradrenergic mechanism causing phasic activity of GnRH neurons and the GABA-mediated synchronous disinhibition of GnRH neurons, causing their synchronous activation, is schematically shown in Fig. 2.

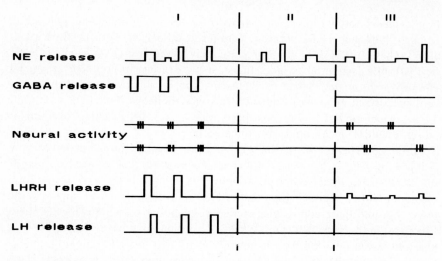

Fig. 2. Schematic considerations of interplay between norepinephrine (*NE*) and GABA to induce phasic and synchronous activation of GnRH neurons. *Panel III* indicates that norepinephrine is necessary to induce phasic activation. It is, however, not able to synchronize the GnRH neurons. For this purpose, a tonic GABAergic inhibition, which prevents the GnRH neurons from phasic activation, is simultaneously relieved (*I*). This results in synchronization of the neurons and bolus-type release of their secretory product, GnRH. Phasic activation of GnRH neurons is prevented when preoptic GABA tonus is constantly high (*Panel II*). (These data summarize results published by Jarry et al. 1990a,b)

Experimental work in the monkey (Gay and Plant 1987), in the rat (Arslan et al. 1988), and on explants of rat hypothalami (Bourguignon et al. 1989a,b) suggests that an excitatory aminoacid neurotransmitter mechanism, which involves the so- called *N*-methyl-D-aspartate (NMDA) receptor may also be involved in inducing pulsatility of GnRH neurons. Systemic injection of the artificial ligand to this receptor, namely NMDA, resulted in prompt release of LH but also of GH, indicating that NMDA causes depolarization of many brain structures. Therefore, this effect may be considered unspecific. Putative endogenous ligands to the NMDA receptors are either glutamate, aspartate, or homocysteic acid. In a previous publication we demonstrated that in the rat preoptic area the release rates of glutamate do not correlate either with pulsatile LH release in ovariectomized rats or in ovariectomized, estrogen-primed rats (Demling et al. 1985). It thus appears that there is no glutamatergic excitatory input to the GnRH neurons. The tonic inhibition and the phasic disinhibition by GABA, however, appear to play an important role in causing their synchronous activation. This conclusion is further justified by our recent demonstration that infusion of GABA into the preoptic area at physiological concentrations, i.e., at doses measured at times of high GABA release rates, has a potent inhibitory action on episodic LH release (Fig. 3; Jarry et al. 1990b).

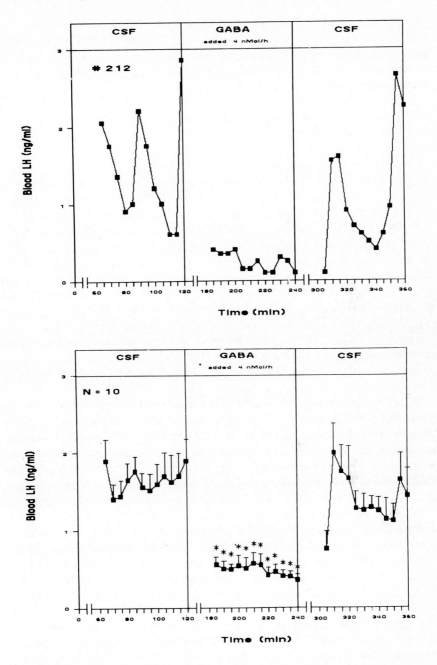

Fig. 3. Infusion of GABA into the preoptic/anterior hypothalamic area in rats results in instantaneous inhibition of pulsatile LH release, indicating that GABA has a strong inhibitory action in the structure where most GnRH perikarya are located. *Upper graph* shows LH levels of an individual animal, *lower graph* details mean values (x+SEM). No such effects were observed when GABA was infused into the mediobasal hypothalamus (data not shown)

With these considerations in mind, we may now address the question of what endogenous opioid peptides, particularly β-endorphin (β-End), might be doing in modulating the pulsatility of the GnRH neurons. Axosomatic as well as axodendritic and dendrodendritic synapses between hypothalamic proopio-melanocortin and GnRH neurons were recently described in the monkey hypothalamus, suggesting direct action of β-End on GnRH neurons (Thind and Goldsmith 1988). Such β-End–GnRH interactions seem to operate also in the rat hypothalamus, for Drouva et al. (1981) showed in vitro a direct inhibitory effect of β-End on potassium-stimulated GnRH release.

It is widely accepted that modulation of LH pulsatility by gonadal steroids involves opioid components. There is overwhelming evidence that the negative feedback action of estradiol (Van Vugt et al. 1982; Bhanot and Wilkinson 1983, 1984; Gabriel et al. 1983; Melis et al. 1984) and of progesterone on LH release is mediated in part via an opioid mechanism (Devorshak- Harvey et al. 1987; Quigley and Yen 1980; Ropert et al. 1981; but see also Babu et al. 1988). Systemic injection of naloxone (an unspecific opiate receptor-blocking drug) into ovariectomized, estrogen-primed rats resulted in a prompt rise in blood LH levels. Furthermore, progesterone, which enhances the negative feedback action of estradiol (Babu et al. 1988), slows down the speed of the pulse generator considerably. This has also been demonstrated in the human (Casper and Alapin-Rubillovitz 1985). This decelerating effect of progesterone on the frequency of the LH pulses was prevented by naloxone, indicating that an endogenous opioid peptide was involved (Quigley and Yen 1980; Ropert et al. 1981).

Little is known about the site of effect of the endogenous opioid peptides. There are two likely locations: at the perikaryal level, which in the rat is the preoptic/anterior hypothalamic area, or at the terminal level of GnRH-containing axons, i.e., at the mediobasal hypothalamus–median eminence complex. Since many of the effects of neurotransmitters are directly exerted at the level of the GnRH perikarya, we decided to utilize the ovariectomized and ovariectomized, estrogen-primed rat implanted with a push-pull cannula in the medial preop-tic/anterior hypothalamic area (Demling et al. 1985; Jarry et al. 1988), and to perfuse this structure with artificial cerebrospinal fluid (CSF) which after 2h was replaced by a β-End-containing CSF solution. After an additional 2-h period, β-End treatment was discontinued and a 2-h CSF control perfusion period ended the experiment. Push-pull perfusion fractions were collected at 5-min intervals and at the end of each fraction period a blood sample was withdrawn through an indwelling catheter in the jugular vein. The same experiments were performed except that instead of β-End, naloxone, a non-specific opiate receptor blocker, was used for perfusion of the preoptic/anterior hypothalamic area. Fig. 4 shows clearly that the high LH levels in ovariec-tomized animals can be reduced by preoptic perfusion of artificial CSF con-taining 10^{-9} M β-End. Measurements from a representative individual animal are also presented in the upper part of Fig. 4, clearly showing that the LH pulsatility observed under CSF control perfusion conditions completely ceased

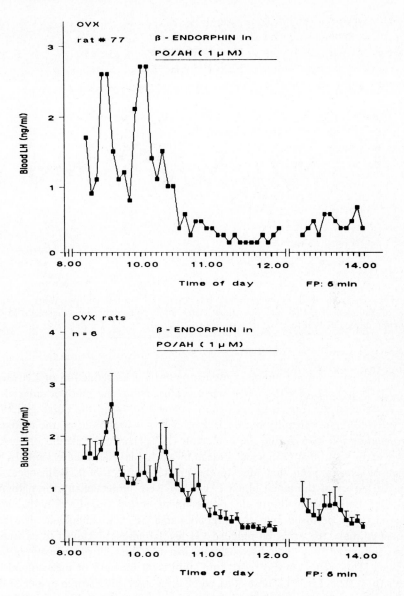

Fig. 4. Infusion of β-End into the preoptic/anterior hypothalamic area of an ovariectomized rat inhibits pulsatile LH secretion, as shown for an individual animal (*upper graph*). This causes significantly decreased mean LH levels (*lower graph*)

during intrapreoptic β-End treatment. It is interesting that the effect of β-End outlasted the remainder of the experiment, which is the reason why mean LH levels remained low in the 2h after β-End treatment. No such effects were observed in ovariectomized, estrogen-primed animals, in which the LH levels were already to a great extent reduced by the estradiol treatment; i.e., preoptic

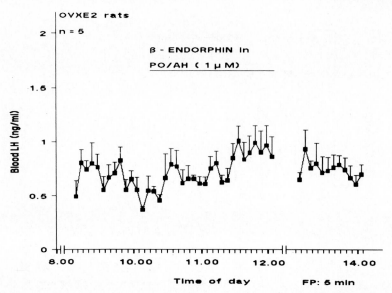

Fig. 5. In ovariectomized, estrogen-primed rats, LH levels are low and pulsatility is largely reduced. Infusion of β-End into the preoptic/anterior hypothalamic area causes no further reduction in mean LH levels)

β-End perfusion did not augment the estrogen-induced reduction of LH levels (Fig. 5). Naloxone (4×10^{-8} M), when perfused into the preoptic area of an ovariectomized rat (Fig. 6 upper panel), seemed to speed the pulse generator up: there were significantly more LH episodes ($p < 0.05$) during the naloxone perfusion period than during the preceding CSF perfusion. This did not result, however, in significantly increased mean blood LH levels in these animals, but it can be clearly seen that, due to the greater number of LH episodes, the standard errors of the mean blood LH levels were larger during the naloxone perfusion period than during the pretreatment period (Fig. 6). Finally, when naloxone was perfused into the preoptic area of ovariectomized, estrogen-primed animals, the estrogen-reduced LH levels increased almost to castration levels and pulsatility, which was virtually absent in the control perfusion period, resumed. This treatment did result in a significant increase of mean blood LH levels ($p < 0.05$, Fig. 7). These data, taken altogether, give strong evidence that β-End acts in the medial preoptic/anterior hypothalamic area. As mentioned earlier, β-End axons form synapses with GnRH neuropil and perikarya. Therefore, it can be speculated that β-End may act directly at these levels on GnRH neurons to reduce either their capability to fire phasically or to interfere with the synchronizing mechanism.

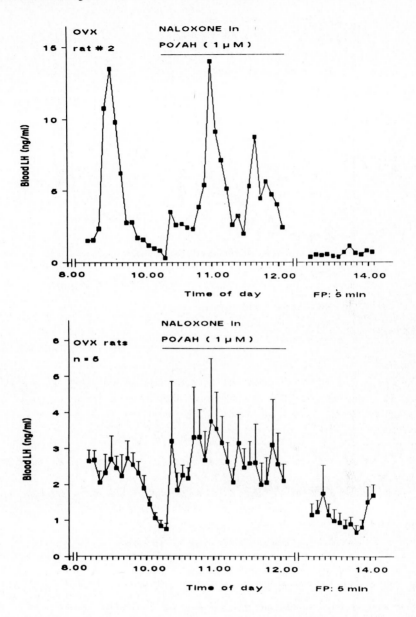

Fig. 6. Infusion of naloxone, an unspecific opiate receptor blocker, into the preoptic/anterior hypothalamic area of ovariectomized rats appears to slightly increase the LH pulse frequency in an individual animal (*upper graph*). The mean LH levels, however, are not significantly increased. The increased pulse frequency seems to increase the standard errors of the means (*lower panel*)

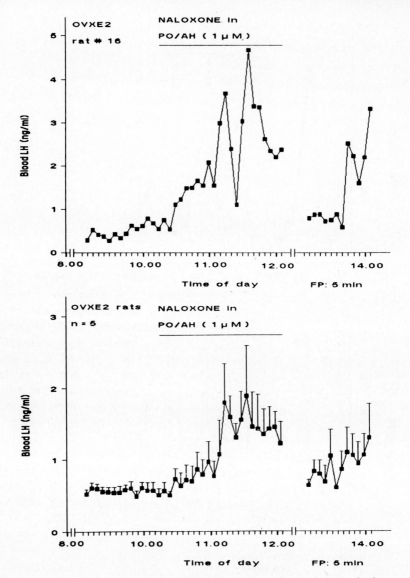

Fig. 7. Preoptic/anterior hypothalamic infusion of naloxone into an ovariectomized, estrogen-primed rat causes immediate recurrence of pulsatile LH release (individual animal, *upper graph*) which results in significantly increased mean LH levels (*lower graph*)

The charm of the push-pull cannula technique is that substances can be applied to a given brain area and that other putative neurotransmitters or peptides, which might be affected by the treatment, can be measured in the effluent push-pull perfusion medium. There is some evidence that opioid peptides act in the hypothalamus via the modulation of a noradrenergic mechanism

Table 1. Concentration of LH in blood and amines in perfusates of the preoptic area ($n = 7$)

	CSF	β-Endorphin	CSF
LH (ng/ml)	1.7 ± 0.4	0.9 ± 0.3[*]	0.9 ± 0.4[*]
Norepinephrine (pg/FP)	4.1 ± 2.9	2.2 ± 1.8[*]	1.8 ± 1.6[*]

mean ± SEM, *$p < 0.05$ vs. CSF.

(Lohse and Wuttke 1981; Kalra and Simpkins 1981). In the following experiments, we analyzed the effluent preoptic push-pull fractions in ovariectomized rats under CSF and β-End perfusion conditions. Fractions were collected at 5-min intervals and norepinephrine, which – as was detailed above – appears to be responsible for phasic activation of GnRH neurons, was measured electrochemically following separation by high-pressure liquid chromatography. Table 1 clearly shows again (like Fig. 4) that during the β-End treatment period mean blood LH levels are decreased. There was a concomitant slight but significant decrease of mean norepinephrine concentrations in the preoptic perfusates during the β-End perfusion period. These changes are very discrete and can be best explained on individual data (Fig. 8). In Figure 8 it is evident that norepinephrine is released in an episodic fashion which does not coincide with LH episodes, indicating again the permissive rather than direct stimulatory effect of norepinephrine on LH release. During the β-End treatment period norepinephrine becomes unmeasurable in many fractions and fewer norepinephrine episodes occurred, this coincided with reduced blood LH levels. During the β-End wash-out period, norepinephrine pulses recur and occasional LH episodes are also observed again. Data reproduced in Table 1 indicate that preoptic release of norepinephrine is indeed statistically significantly reduced during perfusion of this structure with β-End. As mentioned already, the effects of β-End on preoptic norepinephrine release are rather discrete, suggesting that other than noradrenergic, possibly GABAergic, neurons may also be involved in mediating the effects of β-End on GnRH neurons.

In summary, we have reviewed a portion of the literature   and some of our data concerning the role of norepinephrine and GABA in inducing phasic and synchronous activation of GnRH neurons. Norepinephrine must only be present occasionally to induce phasic but asynchronous activation of GnRH neurons. The neurons are then synchronized by simultanous disinhibition of a GABAergic inhibitory tone. This seems to be the basic mechanism for uninfluenced GnRH pulsatility. Endogenous opioid peptides, most likely β-End, are then able to modulate the pulsatility of GnRH neurons, which involves modulation of norepinephrine and possibly also of GABA release. Parts of the steroid feedback of estrogens and progesterone may be explained via the opioid mechanism.

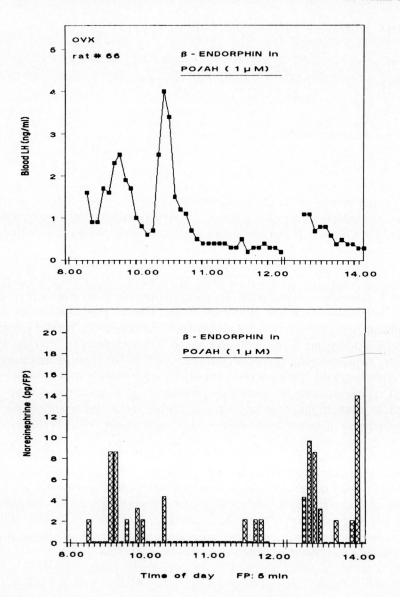

Fig. 8. Infusion of β-End into the preoptic/anterior hypothalamic area of an ovariectomized rat causes reduced pulsatile norepinephrine release in this area. Data of an individual animal are shown in this graph, mean data are summarized in Table 1

References

Arslan M, Pohl CR, Plant TM (1988) DL-2-amino-5-phosphonopentanoic acid, a specific N-methyl-D-aspartic acid receptor antagonist, suppressed pulsatile LH release in the rat. Neuroendocrinology 47: 465-468

Babu GN, Marco J, Bona-Gallo A, Gallo RV (1988) Absence of steroid-dependent, endogenous opioid peptide suppression of pulsatile luteinizing hormone release between diestrus 1 and diestrus 2 in the rat estrous cycle. Neuroendocrinology 47: 249- 258

Bhanot R, Wilkinson M (1983) Opiatergic control of LH secretion is eliminated by gonadectomy. Endocrinology 112: 399-401

Bhanot R, Wilkinson M (1984) The inhibitory effect of opiates on gonadotrophin secretion is dependent upon gonadal steroids. J Endocrinol 102: 133-141

Bourguignon JP, Gerard A, Franchimont P (1989a) Direct activation of gonadotropin-releasing hormone secretion through different receptors to neuroexcitatory amino acids. Neuroendocrinology 49: 402-408

Bourguignon JP, Gerard A, Mathieu J, Simons J, Franchimont P (1989b) Pulsatile release of gonadotropin-releasing hormone from hypothalamic explants is restrained by blockade of N- methyl-D,L-aspartate receptors. Endocrinology 125(2): 1090- 1096

Casper RF, Alapin-Rubillovitz S (1985) Progestins increase endogenous opioid peptide activity in postmenopausal women. J Clin Endocrinol Metab 60: 34-36

Condon TP, Ronnekleiv OK, Kelly MJ (1989) Estrogen modulation of the α-1-adrenergic response of hypothalamic neurons. Neuroendocrinology 50: 51-58

Cooper KJ, Fawcett CP, McCann SM (1973) Variations in pituitary responsiveness to luteinizing hormone releasing factor during the rat estrous cycle. J Endocrinol 57: 187

Crowley WF Jr, Filicori M, Spratt D, Santoro N (1985) The physiology of gonadotropin-releasing hormone (GnRH) secretion in men and women. Recent Prog Horm Res 41: 473

Day TA, Ferguson AV, Renaud LP (1985) Noradrenergic afferents facilitate the activity of tuberoinfundibular neurons of the hypothalamic paraventricular nucleus. Neuroendocrinology 41: 17- 22

Demling J, Fuchs E, Baumert M, Wuttke W (1985) Preoptic catecholamine, GABA and glutamate release in ovariectomized and ovariectomized estrogen-primed rats utilizing a push-pull cannula technique. Neuroendocrinology 41: 212-218

Devorshak-Harvey E, Bona-Gallo A, Gallo RV (1987) Endogenous opioid peptide regulation of pulsatile luteinizing hormone secretion during pregnancy in the rat. Neuroendocrinology 46: 369-378

Drouva SV, Epelbaum J, Tapia-Arancibia L, Laplante E, Kordon C (1981) Opiate receptors modulate LHRH and SRIF release from mediobasal hypothalamic neurons. Neuroendocrinology 32: 163-167

Fox SR, Smith MS (1985) Changes in the pulsatile pattern of luteinizing hormone secretion during the rat estrous cycle. Endocrinology 116(4): 1485-1492

Gabriel SM, Simpkins JW, Kalra SP (1983) Modulation of endogenous opioid influence on luteinizing hormone secretion by progesterone and estrogen. Endocrinology 113(5): 1806-1811

Gay VL, Plant TM (1987) N-methyl-D, L-aspartate elicits hypothalamic gonadotropin-releasing hormone release in prepubertal male rhesus monkeys (Macaca mulatta). Endocrinology 120(6): 2289-2296

Jarry H, Perschl A, Wuttke W (1988) Further evidence that preoptic anterior hypothalamic GABAergic neurons are part of the GnRH pulse and surge generator. Acta Endocrinol (Copenh) 118: 573-579

Jarry H, Leonhardt S, Wuttke W (1990a) A norepinephrine dependent mechanism in the preoptic/anterior hypothalamic area but not in the mediobasal hypothalamus is involved in the regulation of the GnRH pulse generator in ovariectomized rats. Neuroendocrinology 51: 337-344

Jarry H, Leonhardt S, Wuttke W (1990b) Gamma-aminobutyric acid neurons in the preop-
    tic/anterior hypothalamic area synchronize the phasic activity of the GnRH pulse gener-
    ator in ovariectomized rats. Neuroendocrinology (in press)
Kalra SP, Simpkins JW (1981) Evidence for noradrenergic mediation of opioid effects on
    luteinizing hormone secretion. Endocrinology 109: 776-782
Kaufman J-M, Kesner JS, Wilson RC, Knobil E (1985) Electrophysiological manifestation
    of luteinizing hormone- releasing hormone pulse generator activity in the rhesus monkey:
    influence of α-adrenergic and dopaminergic blocking agents. Endocrinology 116: 1327-
    1333
Knobil E (1980) The neuroendocrine control of the menstrual cycle. Recent Prog Horm Res
    36: 53
Leyendecker G, Wildt L (1983) Induction of ovulation with chronic-intermittent (pulsatile)
    administration of GnRH in women with hypothalamic amenorrhea. J Reprod Fertil 69:
    397
Lohse M, Wuttke W (1981) Release and synthesis rate of catecholamines in hypothalamic,
    limbic and midbrain structures following intraventricular injection of β-endorphin in male
    rats. Brain Res 229: 389-402
Melis GB, Paoletti AM, Gambacciani M, Mais V, Fioretti P (1984) Evidence that estrogens
    inhibit LH secretion through opioids in postmenopausal women using naloxone. Neuroen-
    docrinology 39: 60-63
Melrose P, Gross L, Cruse I, Rush M (1987) Isolated gonadotropin- releasing hormone
    neurons harvested from adult male rats secrete biologically active neuropeptide in a
    regular repetitive manner. Endocrinology 121(1): 182-189
Quigley ME, Yen SSC (1980) The role of endogenous opiates on LH secretion during the
    menstrual cycle. J Clin Endocrinol Metab 51: 179-181
Rasmussen DD (1986) Physiological interactions of the basic rest–activity cycle of the brain:
    pulsatile luteinizing hormone secretion as a model. Psychoneuroendocrinology 11(4):
    389-405
Ropert JF, Quigley ME, Yen SSC (1981) Endogenous opiates modulate pulsatile luteinizing
    hormone release in humans. J Clin Endocrinol Metab 52: 583-585
Thind KK, Goldsmith PC (1988) Infundibular gonadotropin-releasing hormone neurons are
    inhibited by direct opioid and autoregulatory synapses in juvenile monkeys. Neuroen-
    docrinology 47: 203-216
Van Vugt DA, Sylvester PW, Aylsworth CF, Meites J (1982) Counteraction of gonadal steroid
    inhibition of luteinizing hormone release by naloxone. Neuroendocrinology 34: 274-278

CRH Inhibition of Gonadotropin and Oxytocin Release: Role of Endogenous Opioids

O.F.X. ALMEIDA

Introduction

It is often forgotten that an organism's response to stressful stimuli may actually be of long-term advantage to the organism itself and/or to its species as a whole. Our negative view of stress is easily understood when one considers that fertility, parturition, and lactation are acutely sensitive to stressors. The disruption of these processes by stress was recorded by Selye (1950) and Cross (1955); these early reports are supported by numerous others — scientific, clinical, and anecdotal. However, it is perhaps only maladaptation to stress that produces undesirable effects on reproduction. The advantages of the stress response are that it ensures that conception, birth, and milk-ejection do not occur at times when the organism's internal environment cannot adequately support these processes, or when its external environment may be hostile to the survival of both mother and young.

The response to stress ultimately involves activation of the hypothalamo-pituitary-adrenal axis; stressors perceived in brain cortical centres result in an increased secretion of hypothalamic corticotropin-releasing hormone (CRH), pituitary adrenocorticotropin (ACTH), and adrenal glucocorticoids (Ganong et al. 1987). It has recently become apparent however, that not all the anti-reproductive effects of stress are caused by elevated adrenal steroid levels; CRH itself is able to act within the hypothalamus to suppress the release of gonadotropin-releasing hormone (GnRH) and, therefore, luteinizing hormone (LH); in addition, it seems that CRH can alter the activity of hypothalamic oxytocinergic neurons, thereby influencing parturition and lactation.

CRH is a peptide comprising of 41 amino acid residues; the amino acid sequence of CRH in humans and rats is identical, and there is a relatively high degree of homology between the sequences of other species. Within the hypothalamus, the peptide is principally synthesized in the parvocellular part of the paraventricular nucleus (PVN), from which fibers are sent to many hypothalamic and extrahypothalamic sites. Some of these fibers terminate in the preoptic area of the hypothalamus where they synapse with GnRH neurons (Leranth et al. 1988); others synapse with proopiomelanocortin-(POMC)-immunoreactive cells in the arcuate nucleus (Hassan et al. 1989).

Until recently, the chief actions of CRH have been thought to be the stimulation of synthesis and release of ACTH from the anterior pituitary; since ACTH and β-endorphin (β-End) are contained in a single prohormone (POMC), changes in ACTH synthesis and release are usually paralleled by changes in β-End, although the latter is subject to several post-translational modifications (Ganong et al. 1987). It is now known that CRH is involved in the integration of a wide variety of behaviors (e.g. locomotion, grooming) and autonomic functions (see Lenz 1988). In addition, CRH stimulates β-End release from the hypothalamus, as well as that of the other two major opioid peptides, dynorphin (Dyn) and methionine-enkephalin (Met-Enk) (Nikolarakis et al. 1986a, 1989). The endogenous opioid peptides (EOP) inhibit gonadotropin (see other chapters in this volume) and oxytocin (OT) (Leng and Russell 1989) secretion. The observation that CRH releases hypothalamic EOP provides an import-ant argument in favor of the idea proposed in the next section, namely, that EOP mediate most of the inhibitory actions of CRH upon LH and OT secretion.

EOP Link in LH-Suppressive Actions of CRH

Rivier and Vale (1984) first showed that CRH produces an inhibition of LH secretion in rats. The same group later demonstrated that administration of an antagonist analogue of CRH could prevent stress-induced reductions in circulating LH levels (Rivier et al. 1986). CRH-evoked increases in glucocorticoid secretion best explained these results (Rivier and Vale 1985). However, the results of studies by our group (Nikolarakis et al. 1986b) suggested that CRH acts within the hypothalamus itself to suppress LH secretion, since CRH was found to be a potent inhibitor of GnRH efflux from rat hypothalami perifused in vitro. Furthermore, Xiao et al. (1989) have recently shown that while glucocorticoids "protect" the female monkey against the LH-inhibitory actions of CRH, these steroids do not mediate the antireproductive effects of CRH; the latter view is also supported by data obtained in women by Barbarino et al. (1989). Central actions of CRH upon GnRH release were indeed suggested by Sirinathsinghji, who observed that CRH inhibited GnRH-dependent sexual behavior when injected into the medial-central gray area of the female rat brain (for review of CRH effects upon sexual behavior, see Almeida et al. 1989).

At the time of our initial studies, the morphological evidence for CRH–GnRH interactions referred to earlier had not been made. In view of (a) Sirinathsinghji's findings that EOP may be involved in the CRH effects upon sexual behavior, (b) evidence that CRH stimulates the secretion of POMC-derived peptides from the pituitary, and (c) the knowledge that EOP inhibit LH secretion by inhibiting GnRH neurons, we pursued the idea that EOP might also mediate the inhibitory actions of CRH upon GnRH release from the hypothalamus. Our observation that CRH stimulated hypothalamic EOP release lent further support to this idea.

The in vivo evidence (Almeida et al. 1988a; Nikolarakis et al. 1989a; Petraglia et al. 1988) that EOP mediate most of the LH-suppressive actions of CRH is:

1. That acute and chronic blockade of EOP receptors with naloxone markedly attenuates the fall in serum LH levels seen after an acute central injection of CRH
2. That pretreatment with an antibody recognizing the N-terminus common to all EOP reduces the depression of LH concentrations caused by CRH
3. That the fall in serum LH levels produced by stress can be partly overcome by the coadministration of antibodies directed against β-End, Dyn and Met-Enk
4. That long-term castrated male rats, which show a subsensitivity to the LH-suppressing effects of opiates such as morphine, are also insensitive to the effects of CRH
5. That morphine-tolerant rats fail to show reductions in their blood LH levels in response to CRH treatment.

The most convincing data for EOP mediation of the CRH effects, however, was provided by experiments with the CRH receptor antagonist, α-helical CRH_{9-41}. In in vivo push-pull (into the mediobasal hypothalamus) and in vitro hypothalamic perfusion experiments, the antagonist produced, concurrently, an increase in GnRH release and a decrease in the release of β-End, Dyn and Met-Enk (Nikolarakis et al. 1988b). These results implied that CRH normally exerts a tonic stimulatory influence upon EOP neurons and, thus, a tonic inhibitory influence upon GnRH and LH secretion. This interpretation is consistent with the now generally accepted view that EOP tonically suppress GnRH neuronal activity (see other chapters in this volume). Of greater interest however, is that the results also suggest that CRH may be of physiological significance to the regulation of GnRH-LH secretion in situations other than stressful ones.

Although Barbarino et al. (1989) found that naloxone pretreatment abolishes the LH-suppressive effects of CRH in women, an analysis of results obtained in our laboratory indicate that EOP mediate only some 70%-80% of the actions of CRH upon LH secretion. While this may be an underestimate, resulting from limitations of the particular manipulations used, it should be recalled that there is morphological evidence for direct CRH-GnRH synaptic connections in the hypothalamus (Leranth et al. 1988) and, in addition, there may well exist other intervening (inhibitory) neurotransmitter/peptidergic systems. The latter suggestion arises from observations that CRH is generally, though not exclusively, an excitatory neuropeptide (Siggins et al. 1985). The relative contribution of one or all of these possible pathways probably varies with the species and sex (cf. Barbarino et al. 1989) and with the prevailing physiological state. The particular opioid mediating the actions of CRH may also be determined by preexisting physiological conditions (including sex hormone status). In the case of footshock stress, however, it seems that β-End may be more important than Dyn which, itself, seems to play a more dominant role than Met-Enk (Petraglia et al. 1988). Although the generality of this rank order remains to be established, it is interesting that the results of other studies show a role for $\mu > \kappa > \delta$ opioid receptors in the regulation of LH secretion in non-stressed rats (Almeida et al. 1988b; Pfeiffer and Pfeiffer, this volume); these findings correspond to the greater affinity of μ-receptors for β-End, of κ-receptors for Dyn, and of δ-receptors for Met-Enk.

CRH and EOP Regulation of Oxytocin Secretion

Central EOP are now regarded as major regulators of parturition and lactation. They exert their effects by inhibiting the secretion of OT, which is essential for stimulating contractions of the myoepithelial cells in the uterus and mammary gland to expel the fetus and to eject milk, respectively. Although still a subject of some controversy, it seems that EOP act at both post-and presynaptic sites of the OT neuron, i.e., upon OT cell bodies in the magnocellular divisions of the hypothalamic supraoptic nucleus (SON) and PVN, and OT terminals in the neurohypophysis, respectively. Existing evidence indicates that μ-and δ-EOP ligands act at postsynaptic sites (Wakerley et al. 1983), whereas κ-ligands act at presynaptic sites (Bicknell and Zhao 1989).

Considerably more is known about the presynaptic opioid regulation of OT secretion than about opioid actions at OT cell bodies. As already mentioned, Dyn seems to be the endogenous ligand responsible for the former. Recent studies have shown that Dyn reaches the OT terminals rather indirectly: the opioid is synthesized in hypothalamic magnocellular neurons which are best known for their production of another neuropeptide, arginine vasopressin (AVP). These neurons also send fibers to the neurohypophysis, where AVP and DYN are coreleased. The opioid apparently interacts directly with κ-opioid receptors on OT terminals, as well as with κ-receptors located on pituicytes (see Bicknell and Zhao 1989). The way in which pituicyte opioid receptor activation results in inhibiton of OT release is thought to involve "envelopment" of the OT terminals by the pituicytes. Thus, EOP control of OT terminal secretion, and ultimately parturition and milk ejection, seems to be coupled to the mechanisms regulating AVP secretion. Osmotic stimuli (which must be of particular relevance during pregnancy and lactation when there are major changes in the salt and water metabolism of the mother) modulate AVP release but, in addition, AVP release is also influenced by EOP (see Summy-Long 1989). At present the interactions between the AVP–EOP–OT systems are not clear. Our understanding of them is further complicated by the fact that almost all stressors stimulate OT secretion, whereas AVP secretion is apparently only altered by osmotic stress. One must, in the meantime, postulate the existence of other mechanisms which prevent births and milk ejections at impropitious times; these very likely involve post-synaptic inhibition by endogenous opioids.

What might be the role of CRH in the control of parturition and lactation ? The answer to this question is still far from clear, although, in view of the central role of CRH in the integration of the stress response and its known stimulatory actions upon hypothalamic EOP release, one would expect it to inhibit OT secretion. Indeed, we observed that central injections of CRH (0.2 nmol) to concious lactating rats reduced the passage of milk to the young by some 80% (Almeida, unpublished data). Although this effect was not reversed by subcutaneous injections of naloxone, we cannot, at present, categorically discount an involvement of EOP since (a) the CRH treatment produced a marked behavioral activation in the mothers; this may have interfered with the nesting and other maternal behaviors prerequisite for milk let-down; (b) naloxone also elicited hyperlocomotion that may have confounded the results in a way similar to that proposed for the CRH effects; and (c) naloxone inhibits the secretion of prolactin which plays an essential role in integrating maternal behaviors. New experiments in which some of these interfering factors can be better controlled (e.g., central injection of drugs into localized brain areas) are necessary before the mechanisms underlying our observations can be defined. It should be pointed out that lactational studies require great care in their performance and interpretation — for instance, concious animals are extremely sensitive to disturbance—and the responses of anesthetized animals are affected by the dehydrating effects of most of the anesthetics used (e.g., urethane), which ultimately alter AVP release. Given these complications, it may not be surprising that recent electrophysiological recordings from anesthetized lactating rats yielded data opposite to those obtained by us: central CRH injections facilitated, rather than depressed, OT cell firing (C.D. Ingram, personal communication).

So far, no studies have investigated the effects of CRH in the control of parturition. However, given the similarities between the neural pathways responsible for eliciting OT secretion in both processes, and the fact that the OT involved in them has a common source, it seems highly probable that CRH regulates parturition via the same mechanisms involved in its control of milk ejection.

Epilogue

Studies of how CRH and EOP interfere with gonadotropin and OT secretion are beginning to provide some insight into how the well-known deleterious effects of stress upon reproductive function might arise. Although still in their infancy, these basic studies may ultimately lead to the development of methods to ensure that the initial response to stress (which has major benefits for the survival of the individual and its species) does not result in a prolonged inhibition of reproductive functions.

Acknowledgements. I wish to thank my collaborators for participation in many of the studies reported here, and the Deutsche Forschungsgemeinschaft (SFB 220) for supporting them.

References

Almeida OFX, Nikolarakis KE, Herz A (1988a) Evidence for the involvement of endogenous opioids in the inhibition of luteinizing hormone by corticotropin-releasing factor. Endocrinology 122: 1034-1041

Almeida OFX, Nikolarakis KE, Webley GE, Herz A (1988b) Opioid components of the clockwork that governs luteinizing hormone and prolactin release in male rats. FASEB J 2: 2874-2877

Almeida OFX, Nikolarakis KE, Sirinathsinghji DJS, Herz A (1989) Opioid-mediated inhibition of sexual behaviour and luteinizing hormone secretion by corticotropin-releasing hormone. In: Dyer RG, Bicknell RJ (eds) Brain opioid systems in reproduction. Oxford University Press, Oxford, pp 149-164

Barbarino A, DeMarinis L, Tofani A, della Casa S, d'Amico C, Mancini A, Corsello SM, Sciuto R, Barini A (1989) Corticotropin- releasing hormone inhibition of gonadotropin release and the effect of opioid blockade. J Clin Endocrinol Metab 68: 523-528

Bicknell RJ, Zhao B-G (1989) Secretory terminals of oxytocin release as a site of opioid modulation. In: Dyer RG, Bicknell RJ (eds) Brain opioid systems in reproduction. Oxford University Press, Oxford, pp 285-307

Cross BA (1955) Neurohormonal mechanisms in emotional inhibition of milk ejection. J Endocrinol 12: 29-37

Ganong WF, Dallman MF, Roberts JL (eds) (1987) The hypothalamic–pituitary–adrenal axis revisited. Ann NY Acad Sci 512: 1-420

Hassan AHS, Almeida OFX, Forgas-Moya l, Gramsch C, Herz A (1989) Immunocytochemical detection of opioid receptors, opioid peptides, and corticotropin-releasing hormone in rat brain and NG108-15 cells. Adv Biosci 75: 293-296

Leng G, Russell JA (1989) Opioids, oxytocin, and parturition. In: Dyer RG, Bicknell RJ (eds) Brain opioid systems in reproduction. Oxford University Press, Oxford, pp 231-255

Lenz HJ (1987) Extrapituitary effects of corticotropin-releasing factor. Hormone & Metabolic Research, Suppl. 16: 17-23

Leranth C, MacLusky NJ, Shanabrough M, Naftolin F (1988) Immunohistochemical evidence for synaptic connections between proopiomelanocortin-immunoreactive axons and LHRH neurons in the preoptic area of the rat brain. Brain Research 449: 167-176

MacLusky NJ, Naftolin F, Leranth C (1988) Immunocytochemical evidence for direct synaptic connections between corticotropin-releasing factor (CRF) and gonadotropin-releasing hormone (GnRH)-containing neurons in the preoptic area of the rat. Brain Res 439: 391-395

Nikolarakis KE, Almeida OFX, Herz A (1986a) Stimulation of hypothalamic β-endorphin and dynorphin release by corticotropin-releasing factor (in vitro). Brain Res 399: 152-155

Nikolarakis KE, Almeida OFX, Herz A (1986b) Corticotropin- releasing factor (CRF) inhibits gonadotropin-releasing hormone (GnRH) release from superfused rat hypothalami in vitro. Brain Res 377: 388-390

Nikolarakis KE, Almeida OFX, Herz A (1988a) Hypothalamic opioid receptors mediate the inhibitory action of corticotropin-releasing hormone on luteinizing hormone release: further evidence from a morphine-tolerant animal model. Brain Res 450: 360-363

Nikolarakis KE, Almeida OFX, Sirinathsinghji DJS, Herz A (1988b) Concomitant changes in the in vitro and in vivo release of opioid peptides and luteinizing hormone-releasing hormone from the hypothalamus following blockade of receptors for corticotropin-releasing factor. Neuroendocrinology 47: 545-550

Nikolarakis KE, Almeida OFX, Herz A (1989) Multiple factors influencing the in vitro release of [Met^5]-enkephalin from rat hypothalamic slices. J Neurochem 52: 428-432

Petraglia F, Vale W, Rivier C (1988) Opioids act centrally to modulate stress-induced decrease in luteinizing hormone in the rat. Endocrinology 119: 2445-2450

Rivier C, Vale W (1984) Influence of corticotropin-releasing factor on reproductive functions in the rat. Endocrinology 114: 914-921

Rivier C, Vale W (1985) Effect of the long-term administration of corticotropin-releasing factor on the pituitary-adrenal and pituitary-gonadal axis in the male rat. J Clin Invest 75: 689-694

Rivier C, Rivier J, Vale W (1986) Stress-induced inhibition of reproductive functions: role of endogenous corticotropin-releasing factor. Science 231: 607-609

Selye H (1950) Stress. Acta, Montreal

Siggins GR, Gruol D, Aldenhof J, Pittman Q (1985) Electrophysiological actions of corticotropin-releasing factor in the central nervous system. Fed Proc 44: 237-242

Sirinathsinghji DJS (1985) Modulation of lordosis behaviour in the female rat by corticotropin releasing factor, β-endorphin and gonadotropin releasing hormone in the mesencephalic central gray. Brain Research 336: 45-55

Summy-Long JY (1989) Cross-inhibition of oxytocin neurons during activation of the vasopressin system. In: Dyer RG, Bicknell RJ (eds) Brain opioid systems in reproduction. Oxford University Press, Oxford, pp 271-284

Wakerley JB, Noble R, Clarke G (1983) Effects of morphine and D-Ala-D-Leu enkephalin on the electrical activity of supraoptic neurosecretory cells in vitro. Neuroscience 10: 73-81

Xiao E, Luckhaus J, Niemann W, Ferin M (1989) Acute inhibition of gonadotropin secretion by corticotropin-releasing hormone in the primate: are the adrenal glands involved? Endocrinology 124: 1632-1637

Differential Role of μ- and κ-Opiate Receptors in Anterior Pituitary Hormone Secretion

D.G. PFEIFFER and A. PFEIFFER

Introduction

Morphine and other opioids are known to affect the release of most anterior pituitary hormones. These actions are thought to be mediated by an interaction with hypothalamic factors which are secreted into the hypothalamo-pituitary circulation (for review see Illes 1989; Pfeiffer and Herz 1984; Millan and Herz 1985). The presence of at least three distinct types of opiate receptors named μ (my), δ (delta) and κ (kappa) is generally accepted and ligands which selectively activate or block these receptors are now available. The existence of several distinct subtypes of opiate receptors not only adds another level of complexity to the analysis of opioid systems; it also raises the question whether there may exist particular physiological functions of, for example, μ- or κ-opiate receptors. In this case, it may become possible to selectively manipulate certain aspects of the endocrine function of opioids.

This review briefly summarizes our studies, which provide some evidence for the involvement of particular types of opiate receptors in the secretion of gonadotropins, prolactin, growth hormone and adrenocorticotropin (ACTH) in rats and in humans. We will also describe studies on the consequences of chronic blockade of endogenous opioids for fecundity and cyclicity in rats.

Luteinizing Hormone and Follicle Stimulating Hormone

Morphine-like opioids were shown to inhibit the release of luteinizing hormone (LH) and to block the preovulatory surge of LH and subsequent ovulation in rats. Opiate antagonists, on the other hand, stimulate the secretion of LH in female and male rats (Bruni et al. 1977) and humans (Quigley and Yen 1980), which suggests a tonic inhibition of LH release by endogenous opioids. The stimulation of LH secretion by opioid antagonists is variable and appears to depend on the steroidal milieu in sexually mature animals and humans (Cicero et al. 1979); for example, in women the effects of opiate antagonists are greatest when estrogen levels are high (Quigley and Yen 1980).

Opioids seem to act at the hypothalamic level by inhibiting the release of luteinizing hormone releasing hormone (LHRH) (Ching 1983). This can be demonstrated in vitro by measuring the inhibition of LHRH release by endogenous and exogenous opioids in isolated hypothalami. This inhibition depends on the levels of testosterone in male rats (Nikolarakis et al. 1986).

For investigating the role of different types of opiate receptors in the release of gonadotropins we used female ovariectomized rats which were implanted with jugular catheters. These catheters were led out of the cages to allow injection of drugs and withdrawal of blood samples without disturbing the animals. The rats were also stereotactically implanted with guide cannulas into the cerebral ventricles for central injection of opioid peptides. The role of different receptors was tested by injecting selective agonists and antagonists at μ- or κ-receptors. In these experiments, a potent and highly selective μ-agonist, [D-Ala^2, MePhe^4, Gly-ol] enkephalin, abbreviated DAGO, potently inhibited LH secretion and its effect was antagonized by either the classical opiate antagonist, naloxone, or by an irreversible and selective μ-receptor antagonist,

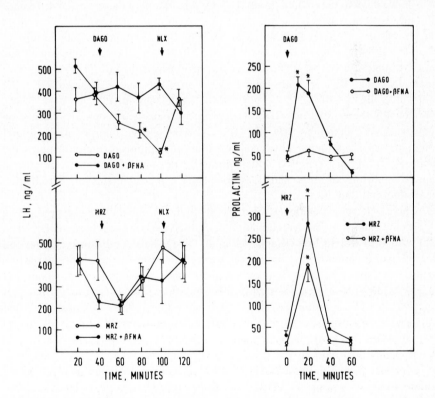

Fig. 1. Effects of the μ-agonist DAGO (1 nmol) and of the κ-agonist MRZ 2549 (*MRZ*, 10 nmol) on the release of LH (*left panel*) and of PRL (*right panel*) in rats (*n* = 5 – 7). The drugs were injected into the lateral cerebral ventricles (i.c.v. 4 μl) and blood was withdrawn through indwelling chronic catheters. To demonstrate an involvement of μ-receptors, rats were treated with the irreversible and selective μ-receptor antagonist β-FNA 4-6 h prior to injection of the opioid. Naloxone (1 mg/kg) was injected i.v. 60 min after the opioid

β-funaltrexamine (Fig.1; Ward et al. 1982). The μ-agonists morphine or DAGO did not affect the release of FSH in intact rats (Pfeiffer et al. 1987).

Further experiments were performed in isolated hypothalami of intact rats by measuring the release of LHRH. The KCl-stimulated release of LHRH was inhibited by the μ-agonist DAGO, but not by the κ-agonist MRZ 2549. Naloxone, moreover, potently stimulated the release of LHRH, demonstrating inhibitory actions of endogenous opioids in this preparation (Pfeiffer et al. 1987), which confirms that opioid effects on LH secretion are mediated at the hypothalamic level.

If opioids tonically suppress LH secretion, what could be their role? To address this question, we treated normal-cyclic female rats with a high dose (2×10mg/day/n = 11/group or 125 μg/kg/h delivered by osmotic minipumps) of the long-lasting opiate antagonist naltrexone. The cycle length, evaluated by vaginal smears, was 4.7 ± 0.5 days in the control group of 11 rats and 4.7 ± 0.3 days in the treated group. During the treatment there was no difference in body weight between the groups. The preovulatory surge of LH, determined in chronically catheterized rats, was of similar magnitude in both groups of animals. Finally, after at least two cycles of treatment, the rats were mated and after completion of pregnancy, the litter size was counted. The incidence of pregnancy was 85% in both groups and control rats had a mean of 8.2 ± 2.5 pups as compared to 9.2 ± 1.5 pups in the treated group (Pfeiffer et al. 1984). Obviously, there was no effect of chronic blockade of opioid systems on reproductive function in rats. This allows two possible interpretations: either there are reserve systems which can substitute for opioids, or opioids may serve a purely inhibitory function which normally becomes functionally important under conditions of stress but does not play an important role in reproduction under normal conditions.

There is some evidence that stress-induced amenorrhea represents a syndrome caused by an overactivation of endogenous opioids, particularly when not related to weight loss (Blankstein et al. 1981). This condition is also termed hypothalamic amenorrhea, indicating normal function of the pituitary and the genital organs. Treatment with opiate antagonists was reported to elevate LH levels in 30%-50% of women with this syndrome and to restore normal pulsatility of LH secretion. Wildt and Leyendecker (1987) demonstrated that ovulatory menstrual cycles can be reinitiated in women with longstanding hypothalamic amenorrhea by treatment with the orally active and long-acting opiate antagonist naltrexone.

Morphine-like opioids inhibit LH secretion in humans probably also by suppressing the release of LHRH. Several μ-receptor agonists like morphine, FK 33824 and buprenorphine were shown to suppress plasma LH levels in man (for references see Pfeiffer and Herz 1984; Millan and Herz 1985). The κ-agonist MR 2034 was shown to possess approximately 10-fold higher affinity for κ-receptors in human brain as compared to rat brain (Pfeiffer et al. 1981). Although this compound affected the release of ACTH, prolactin, growth hormone (GH), and thyroid-stimulating hormone (TSH) in humans, it had no effect on plasma levels of LH and FSH (Pfeiffer et al. 1986a,b). This strongly suggests that, as in rats, the opioid modulation of LH in humans is controlled predominantly by μ-receptors while κ-receptors do not play an important role.

Some reports described an inhibition of LH release by κ-agonists in rats. Most of the compounds employed were not highly selective for κ-receptors and their involvement was not controlled by using a selective μ-receptor antagonist like β-FNA to exclude crossreactivity with μ-receptors (Pechnik et al. 1985; Leadem and Kalra 1985). However, the highly selective κ-agonist U-50488H also inhibited LH secretion, although less potently than the μ-agonists (Leadem and Yagenova 1987). Thus, at least a minor modulation of LH levels via κ-receptors can be demonstrated using some κ-agonists (like U-50488H) but not when using others (like MR 2034 or MRZ 2549). A possible explanation for this observation may be the existence of κ-receptor subtypes, as has been suggested by several groups previously (Pfeiffer et al. 1981; Attali et al. 1982). However, a definitive classification of opiate receptors and their subtypes will have to await their molecular characterization.

Prolactin

The release of prolactin was found to be powerfully stimulated in rats by both μ- and κ-agonists using awake, freely moving animals as described above. The actions of the μ-agonists, morphine and DAGO, were blocked by intracerebroventricular pretreatment with the selective μ-antagonist β-FNA, which demonstrates a central site of action and confirms an involvement of μ-receptors (Fig.1). The κ-agonist MRZ 2549 also caused a massive release of prolactin after central or peripheral administration, but its action was not blocked by μ-antagonist β-FNA. The nonselective μ- and κ-antagonist MR 2266 however, antagonized the effects of MRZ showing an involvement of opiate receptors.

In humans, the κ-agonist MR 2034 caused a strong stimulation of prolactin release which was completely blocked by naloxone pretreatment (Pfeiffer et al. 1986b). Our data thus suggest that both types of receptors can mediate prolactin release in rats and in humans.

Our data agree with those of Krulich et al. (1986) and several other studies (see Illes 1989) performed in rats, while no data except for the study with MR 2034 (Pfeiffer et al. 1986a) are presently available for actions of κ-agonists in humans.

Growth Hormone

The role of different opiate receptors in the secretion of GH is controversial with regard to the role of κ-agonists. Some κ-agonists, like U-50488H (Krulich et al. 1986) were reported to supress GH secretion while others, like ethylketo-

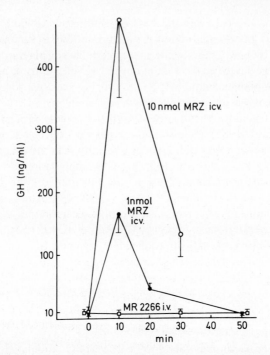

Fig. 2. Effect of the μ-agonist MRZ 2549 (*MRZ*) on plasma GH. Rats were prepared as described in the legend to Fig.1. MR 2266 is a potent opiate receptor antagonist which blocks μ- and κ-receptors

cyclazocine (see Illes 1989) and MRZ 2549 (Fig.2), were potent stimulants of GH release. Again, different types of κ-receptors could play a role here.

Several μ-agonists cause release of GH, while the putative role of δ-receptors needs to be reinvestigated in rats, as discussed comprehensively by Illes (1989). In humans, the κ-agonist MR 2034 was a potent stimulant of GH secretion, which was antagonized by naloxone, demonstrating an involvement of opiate receptors (Pfeiffer et al. 1986a). Since morphine does not release GH in humans, as shown in several studies (see Pfeiffer and Herz 1984), μ-receptors do not appear to be important.

Adrenocorticotropic Hormone

Endogenous opioids are known to inhibit the release of ACTH in rats (Eisenberg 1980) and also in humans (Volavka et al. 1980). This was inferred from a stimulatory effect of naloxone on ACTH and corticosterone or cortisol levels. In rats, the effects of naloxone appear to be mediated centrally, since no effects of opioids or opiate antagonists were observed in pituitary cell preparations, and hypothalamic injection of opioids caused release of ACTH and corticosterone in rats (George and Way 1959; Pfeiffer et al. 1985). At least three neurotransmitters are presently known to affect the release of ACTH from the pituitary: corticotropin releasing hormone (CRH), vasopressin, and catecholamines (Gillies et al. 1982).

The role of CRH in the actions of opioids was investigated by our group using immunoneutralization of CRH. In these experiments rats were pretreated with a specific antiserum to CRH, which neutralized the effect of 0.75 µg CRH administered intravenously. We observed a complete blockade of the stimulatory effect of naloxone on ACTH release (Nikolarakis et al. 1987). The antiserum probably neutralized CRH released by naloxone from the median eminence into the hypothalamo-pituitary circulation. Since opioids are usually inhibitory transmitters, this observation is compatible with a direct inhibitory action of endogenous opioids on CRH release. Since relatively high doses of naloxone are required to obtain an increase in ACTH, it appears most likely that a κ-opiate receptor is involved (Nikolarakis et al. 1987). An involvement of δ-receptors is less likely, because the hypothalamus contains only very low levels of δ-receptors in rats (Goodman et al. 1980) and in humans (Pfeiffer et al. 1982). A recent study reported a direct stimulatory effect of naloxone on the release of CRH from isolated hypothalami in vitro (Tsagarakis et al. 1989).

The actions of exogenous opioids on ACTH release differ between humans and rats. In humans, various µ-receptor agonists inhibit the release of ACTH and cortisol (McDonald et al. 1959; for review see Pfeiffer and Herz 1984). The same is true for the κ-agonist MR 2034 (Pfeiffer et al. 1986b). The receptor involved appears to require high doses of naloxone for antagonism and therefore probably does not represent a typical µ-receptor. The inhibitory actions of the potent µ-agonistic enkephalin derivative FK 33,824 or of morphine cannot be explained by an action at κ-receptors, to which these compounds possess very low affinities. On the other hand, the high dose of naloxone required to antagonize the actions of the κ-agonist MR 2034 is in line with the low affinity of naloxone for κ-receptors in human brain (Pfeiffer et al. 1981). Thus, both µ-and κ-receptors appear to be involved in the opioid regulation of ACTH-release.

In rats, exogenous opioids enhance the release of ACTH by acting at hypothalamic sites (George and Way 1959). The stimulation of either µ- or κ-receptors enhanced the release of ACTH in rats (Fig.3) (Pfeiffer et al. 1985). The actions of κ-receptors were blocked by treatment with an antiserum to CRH, which suggests that pharmacologic stimulation of κ-receptors causes release of CRH in rats (Nikolarakis et al. 1987). The actions of morphine were only partially reduced by pretreatment with the CRH antiserum. However, central µ-receptors, but not κ-receptors, are known to cause a massive release of catecholamines from the adrenal medulla in rats (Pfeiffer et al. 1983), which may release ACTH by stimulation of β-adrenergic receptors in the pituitary. Indeed, a ganglionic blocker also partially reduced the ATCH release caused by morphine. When the ganglionic blocker was combined with the CRH antiserum, the stimulatory effect of morphine was completely blocked (Nikolarakis et al.

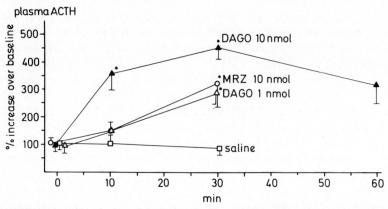

Fig. 3. Effect of the κ-agonist MRZ 2549 (*MRZ*) and of the μ-agonist DAGO on the release of ACTH. Rats were prepared as described in the legend to Fig.1. The data were pooled from several experiments in which baseline levels for ACTH ranged between 40 and 120 pg/ml. Drugs were injected i.c.v. without touching the animals

1989). This indicates that μ-receptor activation in rats releases ACTH by augmenting the central release of CRH and the peripheral release of catecholamines.

The mechanisms by which opioids affect the release of ACTH are highly complex and probably involve at least three separate pathways. Remarkably, studies with isolated hypothalami in which the opioid actions on the release of CRH in rats have been investigated directly suggest that κ-opiate receptors inhibit the release of CRH (Tsagarakis et al. 1989). This contrasts with results obtained in vivo which show a stimulatory action of κ-agonists on the release of ACTH (Pfeiffer et al. 1985, Nikolarakis et al. 1987). At present no explanation for these discrepancies is apparent. Probably, further, as yet unidentified factors also participate in the hypothalamic opioid modulation of the release of ACTH.

References

Attali B, Gouardieres C, Mazarguil H, Audigier Y, Cros J (1982) Evidence for multiple "kappa" binding sites by use of opioid peptides in the guinea pig lumbo-sacral spinal cord. Neuropeptides 3: 53-64

Blankstein J, Reyes FI, Winter JSD, Fairman C (1981) Endorphins and the regulation of the human menstrual cycle. Clin Endocrinol 14: 287-294

Bruni F, van Vugt D, Marshall S, Meites J (1977) Effects of naloxone, morphine and methionine enkephalin on serum prolactin, luteinizing hormone, follicle stimulating hormone, thyroid stimulating hormone and GH. Life Sci 21:461-466

Ching M (1983) Morphine suppresses the proestrous surge of GnRH in pituitary portal plasma of rats. Endocrinology 112: 2209-2211

Cicero TJ, Schainker BA, Meyer ER (1979) Endogenous opioids participate in the regulation of the hypothalamic-pituitary- luteinizing hormone axis and testosterone's negative feedback control of luteinizing hormone. Endocrinology 104: 1286-1291

Eisenberg RM (1980) Effects of naloxone on plasma corticosterone in opiate naive rats. Life Sci 26: 935-943

George R, Way EL (1959) The role of the hypothalamus in pituitary adrenal activation and antidiuresis by morphine. J Pharmacol Exp Ther 125: 111-115

Gillies GE, Linton EA, Lowry PJ (1982) Corticotrophin releasing activity of the new CRF is potentiated several times by vasopressin. Nature 299: 355-357

Goodman RR, Snyder SH, Kuhar MJ, Young WS III (1980) Differentiation of μ-and κ-opiate receptors by light microscopic autoradiography. Proc Natl Acad Sci USA 77: 6239-6242

Illes P (1989) Modulation of transmitter and hormone release by multiple opioid receptors. Rev Physiol Biochem Pharmacol 112: 139-233

Krulich L, Koenig JI, Conway S, McCann SM, Mayfield MA (1986) Opioid κ-receptors and the secretion of PRL and GH in the rat. Neuroendocrinology 99: 411-418.

Leadem CA, Kalra SP (1985) Effects of endogenous opioid peptides and opiates on luteinizing hormone and prolactin secretion in ovariectomized rats. Neuroendocrinology 41: 342-352

Leadem CA, Yagenova SV (1987) Effects of specific activation of μ-, δ and κ-opioid receptors on the secretion of luteinizing hormone and prolactin in ovariectomized rats. Neuroendocrinology 45: 109-117

Linton EA, Tilders FJH, Hodgkinson S, Berkenbosch F, Vermes I, Lowry PJ (1985) Stress induced secretion of corticotrophin is inhibited by antisera to ovine CRF and vasopressin. Endocrinology 116: 966-970

McDonald RK, Evans FT, Weise VK, Patrick RW (1959) Effect of morphine and nalorphine on plasma hydrocortisone levels in man. J Pharmacol Exp Ther 125: 241-247

Millian MJ, Herz A (1985) The endocrinology of the opioids. Int Rev Neurobiol 26: 1-83

Nikolarakis K, Pfeiffer DG, Almeida OFX, Herz A (1986) Opioid modulation of LHRH-release in vitro depends on levels of testosterone in vivo. Neuroendocrinology 44: 314-319

Nikolarakis K, Pfeiffer A, Stalla GK, Herz A (1987) The role of CRF in the release of ACTH by opioid agonists and antagonists in rats. Brain Res 421: 373-376

Nikolarakis K, Pfeiffer A, Stalla GK, Herz A (1989) The role of the sympathetic nervous system and CRH in morphine-stimulated release of ACTH in rats. Brain Res (in press)

Pechnik R, George R, Poland RE (1985) Identification of multiple opiate receptors through neuroendocrine responses. I. Effects of agonists. J Pharmacol Exp Ther 232: 163-169

Pfeiffer A, Pasi A, Mehrain P, Herz A (1981) A subclassification of κ-opiate receptors in human brain by use of dynorphin 1-17. Neuropeptides 2: 87-96

Pfeiffer A, Pasi A, Mehraein P, Herz A (1982) Opiate receptor binding sites in human brain. Brain Res 248: 87-96

Pfeiffer A, Feuerstein G, Zerbe RL, Faden AI, Kopin IJ (1983) μ-Receptors mediate opioid cardiovascular effects at anterior hypothalamic sites through sympatho-adrenomedullary and parasympathetic pathways. Endocrinology 113: 929-938

Pfeiffer A, Herz A (1984) Endocrine actions of opioids. Horm Metab Res 16: 386-397

Pfeiffer A, Herz A, Loriaux DL, Pfeiffer DG (1985) Central κ- and μ- opiate receptors mediate ACTH-release in rats. Endocrinology 116: 2688-2690

Pfeiffer A, Braun S, Mann K, Meyer HD, Brantl V (1986a) Anterior pituitary hormone responses to a κ-opioid agonist in man. J Clin Endocrinol Metab 62: 181-185

Pfeiffer A, Knepel W, Braun S, Meyer HD, Lohmann H, Brantl V (1986b) Effects of a κ-opioid agonist on adrenocorticotropic and diuretic functions in man. Horm Metab Res 18: 842-848

Pfeiffer DG, Nikolarakis K, Pfeiffer A (1984) Chronic blockade of opiate receptors: influence on reproduction and body weight in female rats. Neuropeptides 5: 279-282

Pfeiffer DG, Pfeiffer A, Almeida OFX, Herz A (1987) Opiate suppression of LH secretion involves opiate receptors different from those mediating opiate effects on prolactin secretion. J Endocrinol 114: 469-476

Quigley ME, Yen SSC (1980) The role of endogenous opioids in LH secretion during the menstrual cycle. J Clin Endocrinol Metab 51: 179-181

Stalla GK, Hartwimmer J, Kaliebe T, Müller OA (1985) Radioimmunoassay of human CRF. Acta Endocrinol [Suppl] (Copenh) 267: 108-118
Tsagarakis S, Rees LH, Besser G M, Grossman A (1989) Opiate receptor subtype regulation of CRF-41 release from rat hypothalamus in vitro. Neuroendocrinology (in press)
Volavka J, Baumann J, Pevnick J, Reker D, James B, Cho D (1980) Short term hormonal effects of naloxone in man. Psychoneuroendocrinology 5: 225-234

Peripheral Opioid Secretion

Paracrine Control of Testicular Function: Role of Opioids

J.M.S. BARTLETT

In recent years the study of local hormonal interactions within organs, or paracrinology, as it is properly called, has expanded rapidly. Within many organs complex cell interactions have been described, which appear to occur solely between cells of the organ in question. Of all organs studied in this way perhaps the gonads have received most attention. Many locally produced factors within the testis and ovary have been postulated to exert paracrine actions. However, when studying paracrine interactions within any organ, the importance of peripheral control of cell function should not be forgotten. This is particularly true of the testis. Furthermore, discussions of testicular function must take into account not only endocrine actions on the organ but also the great complexity of testicular structure, which in itself is undoubtably the cause of some of the local interactions observed.

Testicular Structure Function and Pituitary Regulation of Testicular Function

The testis performs a dual role, both as an endocrine organ and as the site of gamete production in the male. The actions of testosterone throughout life are central to the development and maintenance of male characteristics, whilst gamete production is essential for the fathering of offspring. Development of external genetalia and accessory sex organs, hair and bone growth, hemoglobin production, nitrogen balance, libido and erectile potency, muscle development, vocal register, and pysche are dependent on testosterone secretion.

Pituitary gonadotrophins play a central role in the development and maintenance of normal testicular function. Both follicle stimulating hormone (FSH) and luteinizing hormone (LH) are essential for the establishment of normal testicular function. LH acts primarily through the stimulation of testosterone production by Leydig cells within the testis; this testosterone produced by Leydig cells acts within the testis in the initiation and maintenance of spermatogenic function. In some experimental models, it has been proven that testosterone can both initiate and maintain spermatogenesis in the absence of gonadotrophins (Ahmad et al. 1973, 1975; Marshall et al. 1983; 1987; Bartlett et al. 1988b). However, in physiology, FSH is known to play a central role in the initiation of spermatogenesis in man and many animal models (Wickings et al. 1980; Srinath et al. 1983; Marshall et al. 1986; Matsumoto and Bremner 1987; Marshall and Nieschlag 1987; Bartlett et al. 1989).

Testicular Structure and Morphology

The mammalian testis is separated into two major compartments, the avascular seminiferous tubules, which comprise over 80% of the testicular mass in most animals, and the vascularized interstitium which comprises about 16% of the testicular mass and contains the Leydig cells, macrophages, and other minor cell components (Christiansen 1975).

The interstitial and seminiferous compartments of the testis are separated by a dual barrier, firstly at the level of the peritubular myoid and endothelial cells and secondly at the level of the Sertoli cell tight junctions. Between them these barriers provide a functional separation between the testicular interstitium and the tubular lumen which is the sight of gamete production or spermatogenesis (Setchell 1980).

The process of spermatogenesis involves the development of stem cells, spermatogonia, through a number of cell divisions to form haploid spermatids. This process is supported by Sertoli cells both structurally and metabolically. Due to the requirement in the male for a daily output of large numbers of spermatozoa, testicular structure is extremely complex with numerous cell associations existing simultaneously in close proximity in this organ, requiring stringent control of the hormonal environment (see reviews by Sharpe 1982, 1984, 1986; Parvinen 1982, Nieschlag and Bartlett 1989).

Paracrine Interactions Within the Testis

Over recent years the number of paracrine interactions described within the testis has increased dramatically. The complexity of testicular structure appears to require that many factors are produced locally within the seminiferous tubules or within the testicular interstitium. For the purposes of this review it is important to note that, whilst certain roles for opioid peptides have been described within the testis, many factors other than opioids play a major role in the regulation of testicular functions (Parvinen 1982; Sharpe 1982, 1984, 1986, Nieschlag and Bartlett 1989).

Opioid Families

Opioids are produced from precursor molecules which code for several peptides simultaneously. Currently three such precursors are known and these allow the separation of opioids into three subgroups as follows (Howlett and Rees 1987):

1. Proenkaphalin derived peptides: including met-enkephalin, leu- enkephalin, extended forms of met-enkephalin, and peptide E.
2. Prodynorphin derived peptides: including leu-enkephalin, dynorphin, rimorphin, α-neoendorphin and β-neoendorphin.
3. Proopiomelanocortin derived peptides: including β-endorphin, in conjunction with which α-melanocyte-stimulating hormone (MSH), β-lipotropin (β-LPH), and ACTH are also secreted. Some of these nonopioids are also implicated in opioid controlled paracrine interactions and will therefore be included in this discussion where relevant. In addition to β-endorphin a number of β-endorphin metabolites are implicated in testicular regulation to a small degree.

Opioids and Pituitary Function

Opioids have been shown to modulate secretion or synthesis of all pituitary hormones (Meites et al. 1979; Grossman 1983; Morley 1981). The involvement of opioids in regulation of pituitary hormones undoubtably results in changes in peripheral stimulation of testicular function, and these effects complicate the interpretation of in vivo studies of paracrine actions of these substances.

Localization of Genes/Gene Products Within the Testis

Proopiomelanocortin

Evidence for the involvement of peptides derived from the proopiomelanocortin (POMC) molecule in the control of testicular function is growing rapidly, following the discovery of POMC gene transcripts and gene products within the testis. However, as yet, a clear explanation of the role of these peptides within the testis is not forthcoming. Initial findings suggested that the POMC gene was localized in Leydig cells, based on experiments using Leydig cell tumor lines (Chen et al. 1984). Since then the presence of POMC gene transcripts within the testis, not all localized to the Leydig cells, have been widely reported (Engelhardt 1989; Lacaze-Mosmonteil et al. 1987; Kilpatrick et al. 1987; Gizang-Ginsberg and Wolgemuth 1985, 1987; Boitani et al. 1986; Bardin et al. 1984; Chen et al. 1984; Melner and Puett 1984). Many groups report finding of truncated POMC transcripts shorter than the hypothalamic gene product (Lacaze-Mosmonteil et al. 1987; Kilpatrick et al. 1987; Boitani et al. 1986; Bardin et al. 1984). The presence of such truncated transcripts may, in part, account for the apparent reduced efficacy of translation observed (Chen et al. 1984). Alternatively, it has been suggested that these short transcripts, lacking as they do the signal peptide required for membrane translocation and precursor processing, are partially or fully inactive (Lacaze-Mosmonteil et al. 1987). However, the presence of lesser amounts of the normal 1200 nucleotide mRNA species within the testis suggests that authentic POMC can be produced within the testis (Lacaze-Mosmonteil et al. 1987).

Confirmation of the presence of POMC messenger ribonucleic acid (mRNA) in Leydig cells (Gizang-Ginsberg and Wolgemuth 1985, 1987; Boitani et al. 1986; Bardin et al. 1984; Melner and Puett, 1984) has been followed by suggestions that POMC transcripts are also present in spermatocytes and spermatogonia (Kilpatrick et al. 1987; Gizang-Ginsberg and Wolgemuth 1985, 1987), although the low level of signal in some studies (Gizang-Ginsberg and Wolgemuth 1985) and the failure to detect mRNA in others (Bardin et al. 1984) have led to controversy in this area.

POMC gene products have also been demonstrated within the testis, with the first findings coming as early as 1982 (Tsong et al. 1982). It has been suggested that β-endorphin is the major product in the testis, with lesser amounts of α-and γ-endorphin, α-MSH and ACTH being detected (Tsong et al. 1982; Margioris et al. 1983; Boitani et al. 1985; Fabbri et al. 1988). Production of these peptides has been localized to Leydig cells (Margioris et al. 1983; Shaha et al. 1984; Chen et al. 1984, Bardin et al. 1984, Boitani et al. 1985, Fabbri et al. 1988, 1989), with little evidence for localization elsewhere in the testis (Bardin et al. 1984; Boitani et al. 1985). It may be that transcripts in germ cells lack the translation signals required for peptide synthesis. Nevertheless, endorphin-derived molecules have been localized within germ cells (Cheng et al. 1985). The localization of the n-acetyl endorphins is similar to that of γ-endorphin generating peptidase (Lebouille et al. 1986), and it is suggested that these activities represent metabolism of Leydig cell endorphins within the seminiferous tubules.

Testicular production of endorphin has been shown to change in an age-related fashion, with levels rising sharply in rat testes between 20 and 60 days of age from barely detectable levels to levels which remained constant into maturity (Adams and Cicero 1989). Furthermore, with the onset of puberty, a qualitative change in peptide produced occurred, from predominantly β-endorphin from 5 to 15 days, to predominantly β-lipotropin from the onset of puberty (30 days) and thereafter (Adams and Cicero 1989). In adult animals, Leydig cell production of β-endorphin has been shown to be regulated by gonadotrophins, steroids, and gonadotrophin-releasing hormone (GnRH; Fabbri et al. 1989) and stimulation of GnRH production by endorphins may demonstrate a closed loop system for the regulation of endorphin effects in the testis (Engelhardt 1989).

Proenkephalin

Proenkephalin mRNA has been isolated along with low amounts of its gene products in both ovary and testis (Kilpatrick et al. 1985; Douglass et al. 1987), these mRNAs appear to be localized within the seminiferous tubule (Kilpatrick and Rosenthal 1986; Kilpatrick et al. 1987; Yoshikawa and Aizawa 1988b; Yoshikawa et al. 1989a). Despite these findings, enkephalin immunoreactivity is found in both seminiferous tubules and Leydig cells (Engelhardt et al. 1986; Schulze et al. 1987). Also, reports of a large, 1900 bp mRNA which is only poorly translated due to a mutated coding sequence (Kilpatrick et al. 1985) confuse the issue somewhat. In testicular tissues proenkephalin expression is markedly higher than either POMC or prodynorphin mRNAs (Douglass et al. 1987), and two further mRNA transcripts for proenkaphalin have been found, both of differing lengths and longer than the hypothalamic sequence (Kilpatrick et al. 1985; Douglass et al. 1987). No mRNA hybridization for proenkephalin complementary DNA (cDNA) could be found in mouse or rat tumor Leydig cells (McMurray et al. 1989), whilst somatic and germ cell lines do contain these transcripts (Kilpatrick and Milette 1986; Kilpatrick et al. 1987). Furthermore, mRNAs for preproenkephalin, which may not be identical, have been localized within peritubular cells and round spermatids (Yoshikawa et al. 1989a, b). The role of the peritubular cell mRNA, which responds to both cyclic adenosine monophosphate (cAMP) and phorbol esters, in testicular function is not clear (Yoshikawa et al. 1989a). It would now appear that the proenkephalin transcript, which most closely resembles hypothalamic mRNA, is found in Sertoli cells (Kilpatrick et al. 1987). However, the predominant message, of 1700 bp, is localized within pachytene spermatocytes and round spermatids (Kilpatrick and Milette 1986). Furthermore, the ontogeny of this signal, which appears within tubules at a time corresponding with the appearance of round spermatids in puberty, strongly suggests that it plays some role in germ cell development (Engelhardt 1989; Kilpatrick and Milette 1986).

Both immunoreactive met-and leu-enkephalins have been identified within the testis (Kilpatrick et al. 1985; Cox et al. 1987). Their secretion appears to be controlled by gonadotrophins (Saint Pol et al. 1986, 1988), with marked effects of both FSH and human chorionic gonadotrophin (hCG) on Sertoli cell expression of these products (Yoshikawa and Aizawa 1988a; Kew and Kilpatrick 1989). However, paracrine regulation has not been ruled out (Engelhardt 1989). Immunohistochemical staining has shown the presence of enkephalins within spermatogonia in juvenile and adult animals, primary spermatocytes, and Sertoli cells in adults, and in Leydig cells throughout development (Engelhardt et al. 1986). The significance of this latter staining is not clear since proenkephalin mRNA has not yet been identified in Leydig cells (Engelhardt 1989), but it is possible that enkephalins are produced by Leydig cells for paracrine action on seminiferous tubules.

Prodynorphin

Prodynorphin mRNA and immunoreactive dynorphin A and B have also been identified within testicular tissue of rat, rabbit and guinea pig. In all species activity for both peptides was in the femtomolar range (Douglass et al. 1987), suggesting that these factors may also be involved in testicular regulation. More recently, expression of the prodynorphin gene has been found in a Leydig tumor cell line (McMurray et al. 1989). In this cell line, gene products are also detectable at levels similar to those found in whole testis extracts (McMurray et al. 1989; Douglass et al. 1987). Similar to findings for POMC, prodynorphin mRNA levels were increased when cells were exposed to cAMP (McMurray et al. 1989), which suggests that in normal cell lines this gene product may be susceptible to hormonal regulation (McMurray et al. 1989). However, target cells and actions for these peptides in the testis have not yet been demonstrated.

Actions of Opioids

Sertoli Cell Division

The discovery of opioid binding sites within the testis (Boitani et al. 1984), and their subsequent localization to Sertoli cells (Fabbri et al. 1989) has intensified investigations into regulation of Sertoli cell function by opioids. Several studies have provided evidence that β-endorphin inhibits FSH-stimulated Sertoli cell division and other FSH-regulated functions (Orth 1986; Boitani et al. 1985; Gerendai et al. 1986; Fabbri et al. 1989) whilst ACTH and α-MSH act to stimulate cell division and Sertoli cell function (Bardin et al. 1984; Boitani et al. 1986). More recent data suggests that this simplistic antagonism may not be the case since α-MSH, whilst stimulating cAMP production and aromatase activity, inhibits plasminogen activator production in juvenile rat Sertoli cell cultures (Boitani et al. 1988). However, the ontogeny of these effects correlates well with findings on the ontogeny of β-endorphin in the testis which show that before 20 days of age, when Sertoli cell division occurs in the rat, levels of β-endorphin are low, rising between 20 and 60 days of age to adult levels (see above). Therefore it would appear that in early puberty one role of β-endorphin is to regulate in conjunction with FSH and MSH the proliferation of Sertoli cells within the testis. The involvement of other opioid peptides in this mechanisms has not been investigated.

Opioid Regulation of Sertoli Cell Function

In addition to the putative roles of opioids in pubertal development a number of observations suggest that these peptides can modulate Sertoli cell function in other ways, in both pubertal and adult animals. However, in adults the picture is complicated by the presence of large numbers of germ cells in close contact with Sertoli cells which may in themselves modulate Sertoli cell function (see Nieschlag and Bartlett 1989), and by numerous other factors which modulate the effects of gonadotrophin and paracrine hormones.

Both β-endorphin and the enkephalin family have been implicated in the regulation of Sertoli cell function, with some indication in the case of the enkephalins that a paracrine feedback between the Sertoli cell and the Leydig cell may exist. However, knowledge of the possible role of dynorphins in testicular function is lacking at present.

β-Endorphin is known to modulate FSH stimulation of synthetic processes within the Sertoli cell via modulation of adenylate cyclase activity (Morris et al. 1987). The possibility exists that, via this mechanism, β-endorphin modulates all functions of the Sertoli cells which are stimulated by FSH, although as yet only a few specific effects of β-endorphin on Sertoli cell function have been documented — notably on production of androgen binding protein (ABP) and inhibin (Morris et al. 1987; Fabbri et al. 1989). However, the precise physiological role of these modulations of peripheral stimulation by FSH (inhibin) and FSH and androgens (ABP) is not clear. Any interpretation of the effects of opioid peptides in this context must take into account the numerous factors other than β-endorphin that are known to modulate FSH action (Fig 1). FSH enters the testis via the testicular blood supply and binds to specific receptors on the

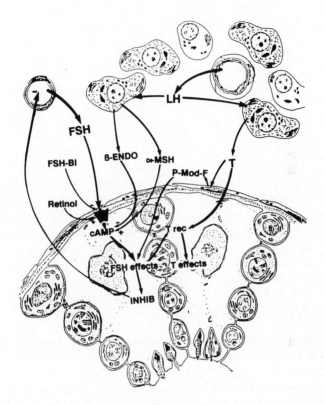

Fig.1. Opioid regulation of FSH action in the testis. β-*ENDO*, β-endorphin; FSH-BI, FSH-binding inhibitor; *P-Mod-F*, peritubular modifying factor; *T*, testosterone; *INHIB*, inhibin; *T rec*, testosterone receptors

Sertoli cell (Marshall and Nieschlag 1987). Two distinct factors are known to affect this step. Vitamin A (retinol) regulates the number of receptors present in Sertoli cells, such that in deficient animals FSH receptor levels are reduced (Unni and Rao 1986). In addition, the existence of an inhibitor of FSH binding to its receptor has also been established (Krishnan et al. 1986). Once FSH is bound to its receptor, activation of adenylate cyclase produces increased levels of the second messenger cyclic AMP, and it is this step which is thought to be regulated by opioids (Morris et al. 1987). However, in addition to these factors, the production of factors from peritubular cells (peritubular modifying factor α and β), under testosterone stimulation, which potentiate FSH action on Sertoli cell functions at a level not yet established (Skinner and Fritz 1985a, b), further complicates the issue. Nor are the actions of modulators of FSH function necessarily limited to FSH effects: since FSH is known to stimulate testosterone receptor levels in Sertoli cells (Verhoeven and Cailleau 1988), it is plausible that modulators of FSH function can also control to a lesser extent the action of testosterone. It can be appreciated, therefore, that the actions of opioid peptides in regulation of testicular function could be both wide ranging and difficult to evaluate, due to the complexity of the system under investigation.

In addition to the factors shown to be regulated by opioid action, ABP and inhibin (Morris et al. 1987; Fabbri et al. 1989), a number of other factors whose synthesis and secretion are regulated by either FSH or, indirectly, testosterone may in future be shown to be affected by the action of opioids. These include FSH-stimulated factors as diverse as plasminogen activator, transferrin, glucose transport, and lactate productio (Bartlett and Nieschlag 1987 for review). In addition, removal of certain germ cell types from the testis also affects production of ABP (Bartlett et al. 1988a), although this effect may be modulated through changes in FSH. However, the presence of γ-endorphin generating peptidase, an enzyme involved in the cleavage of β-endorphin to α and γ-endorphins, and of acetylated forms of endorphin within germ cells (Cheng et al. 1985; Lebouille et al. 1986), may denote that this effect is mediated via other means. With respect to inhibin, both FSH and LH have been shown to stimulate the production of inhibin, and P-mod-F has been shown to modulate the effect of FSH on inhibin production in a positive fashion (Skinner 1989). Since it has now been suggested that both Leydig cells and Sertoli cells produce inhibin and activin (de Jong and Robertson 1985; Tsonis and Sharpe 1986), the overall picture regarding regulation of this hormone within the testis has become markedly more complicated. The physiological role of paracrine regulation of inhibin production, should the role of this hormone relate solely to pituitary FSH production, is unclear. However, the suggestion that inhibin itself may play a paracrine role in germ cell division (van Dissel-Emiliani et al. 1988) and growth factor activities of activin and inhibin (Franchimont et al. 1981; Carson et al. 1988; Hedger et al. 1989) may indicate that the functional role of the inhibin family of hormones is also more complex than hitherto thought.

Despite the complexity of paracrine and endocrine regulation of Sertoli cell function, it is clear that the mechanism by which β-endorphin modulates Sertoli cell function could suggest that this factor plays a key role in the paracrine regulation of FSH action.

The Opioid Closed Loop System Regulating Leydig Cell Function

Amongst the earliest roles suggested for testicular opioids was the regulation of Leydig cell testosterone production (Boitani et al. 1985; Gerendai et al. 1986) although some authors do not show this effect (Sharpe and Cooper 1987). β-Endorphin inhibits LH-stimulated testosterone production by Leydig cells (Boitani et al. 1985; Gerendai et al. 1986; Juniewicz et al. 1988). However, since β-endorphin is merely one of many factors known to modulate Leydig cell testosterone production (reviewed by Sharpe 1982, 1984, 1986; Nieschlag and Bartlett 1989), its role in this instance as an autocrine regulator of testosterone production may be of marginal interest. Of potentially greater interest is the closed loop feedback regulation of β-endorphin and possibly α-MSH, enkephalins and the Sertoli cell LHRH-like peptide, which also plays a minor role in the regulation of testosterone production (Sharpe 1984, 1986).

β-Endorphin production by the Leydig cell is regulated primarily via LH: binding of LH to its receptor on the Leydig cell stimulates production of β-endorphin (Bardin et al. 1984; Fabbri et al. 1989). β-Endorphin is released from the Leydig cell and is then available either to act on the Sertoli cell or to regulate Leydig cell function as described above. Immunoreactive enkephalins, present within germ cells and Leydig cells, are also released into the interstitium (Engelhardt et al 1986; Saint-Pol et al. 1986, 1988; Schulze et al. 1987), from where they too may act upon Sertoli cell receptors for enkephalins (Engelhardt 1989). The production of enkephalins appears to be under the control of LH (Saint-Pol et al. 1986, 1988). It would appear that under stimulation from these enkephalins, with the possible involvement of β-endorphin, the Sertoli cells produce and secrete increased amounts of the testicular LHRH-like factor (Saint Pol et al. 1988). This product in turn acts upon specific Leydig cell LHRH receptors and both modulates steroid production (Sharpe 1986) and inhibits the production of β-endorphin by Leydig cells (Fabbri et al. 1989). The putative involvement of FSH in the stimulation of LHRH may further establish this as a closed loop feedback system of paracrine control between Leydig and Sertoli cells (Fig.2).

Conclusions

Overall it would appear that the understanding of testicular functions of opioids is developing rapidly. It is likely that in the near future further functional roles for the POMC and enkephalin gene products will be identified, and that a role for the dynorphins, which as yet have no known testicular function, will be established. The central position of β-endorphin in the regulation of FSH action suggests that opioids play a central role in testicular function, but the lack of experimental models to date has prevented a conclusive investigation of the role of these peptides in physiology.

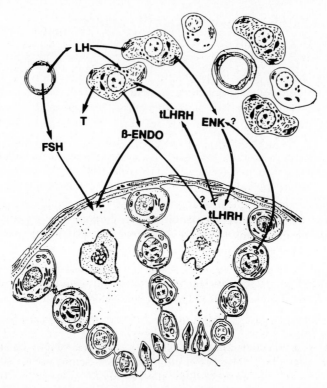

Fig.2. Sertoli cell–Leydig cell regulation via opioid peptides. β-*ENDO*, β-endorphin; *ENK*, enkephalins; *tLHRH*, testicular LHRH-like factor; *T*, testosterone

References

Adams ML, Cicero TJ (1989) The ontogeny of immunoreactive β-endorphin and β-lipotropin in the rat testis. Life Sci 44 (2): 159-66

Ahmad N, Haltmeyer GC, Eikness KB (1973) Maintenance of spermatogenesis in rats with intratesticular implants containing testosterone or dihydrotestosterone. Biol Reprod 8: 411-419

Ahmad N, Haltmeyer GC, Eikness KB (1975) Maintenance of spermatogenesis in rats with testosterone or dihydrotestosterone in hypophysectomised rats. J Reprod Fertil 44: 103-107

Bardin CW, Shaha C, Mather J, Salomon Y, Margioris AN, Liotta AS, Gerendai I, Chen CL, Krieger DT (1984) Identification and possible function of pro-opiomelanocortir-derived peptides in the testis. Ann NY Acad Sci 438: 346-364

Bartlett JMS, Kerr JB, Sharpe RM (1988a) The selective removal of pachytene spermatocytes using methoxy acetic acid as an approach to the study in vivo of paracrine interactions in the testis. J Androl 9: 31-40

Bartlett JMS, Weinbauer GF, Nieschlag E (1988b) The role of FSH in the maintenance of spermatogenesis. In: Cooke BA, Sharpe RM. (eds) The molecular and cellular endocrinology of the testis. Raven, New York, pp 271-274 (Serono symposia, vol 50)

Bartlett JMS, Weinbauer GF, Nieschlag E (1989) Differential effects of FSH and testosterone on the maintenance of spermatogenesis in the adult hypophysectomised rat. J Endocrinol 121: 49-58

Boitani C, Chen C-L, Canipari R, Bardin CW (1988) Expression of the pro-opiomelanocortin (POMC) gene in rat testicular germ cells and the response of Sertoli cells to POMC-derived peptides. In: Cooke BA, Sharpe RM. (eds) The molecular and cellular endocrinology of the testis. Raven, New York, pp 303-309 (Serono symposia, vol 50)

Boitani C, Chen C-L, Margioris AN, Gerendai I, Morris PL, Bardin CW (1985) Pro-opiomelanocortin-derived peptides in the testis: evidence for a possible role in Leydig and Sertoli cell function. Med Biol 63: 251-258

Boitani C, Mather JP, Bardin CW (1986) Stimulation of adenosine 3',5'-monophosphate production in rat Sertoli cells by alpha- melanotropin-stimulating hormone (alpha MSH) and des-acetyl alpha MSH. Endocrinology 118 (4): 1513-1518

Boitani C, Shaha C, Bardin CW, Hahn EF (1984) Opiate receptor binding in the testis (Abstr 254). In: Proceedings of the 7th International Congress of Endocrinology. Excerpta Medica, Amsterdam

Carson RS, Robertson DM, Findlay JK (1988) Ovine follicular fluid inhibits thymidine incorporation by 3T3 fibroblasts in vitro. J Reprod Fertil 82: 447-455

Chen CL, Mather JP, Morris PL, Bardin CW (1984) Expression of pro-opiomelanocortin-like gene in the testis and epididymis. Proc Natl Acad Sci USA 81 (18): 5672-5675

Cheng MC, Clements JA, Smith AI, Lolait SJ, Funder JW (1985) N-acetyl endorphin in rat spermatogonia and primary spermatocytes. J Clin Invest 75 (3): 832-835

Christiansen AK (1975) Leydig cells. In: Greep RO, Ashwood EB (eds) Handbook of physiology, vol 7. American Physiological Society, Washington, pp 57-94

Cox BM, Rosenberger JG, Douglas J (1987) Chromatographic characterisation of dynorphin and (Leu) enkephalin immunoreactivity in guinea pig and rat testis. Regul Pept 19: 1-12

De Jong FH, Robertson DM (1985) Inhibin: 1985 update on action and purification. Mol Cell Endocrinol 42: 95-103

Douglass J, Cox B, Quinn B, Civelli O, Herbert E (1987) Expression of the prodynorphin gene in male and female mammalian reproductive tissues. Endocrinology 120: 707-713

Engelhardt RP (1989) Opioïdes gonadiques et fonction testiculaire. Ann Endocrinol (Paris) 50 (1): 64-72

Engelhardt RP, Saint-Pol P, Tramu G, Leonardelli J (1986) Immunohistochemical localization of enkephalinlike peptides during testicular development in rats. Arch Androl 17 (1): 49-56

Fabbri A, Jannini EA, Gnessi L, Ulisse S, Moretti C, Isidori A (1989) Neuroendocrine control of male reproductive function. The opioid system as a model of control at multiple sites. J Steroid Biochem 32 (1B): 145-50

Fabbri A, Knox G, Buczko E, Dufau ML (1988) β- endorphin production by the fetal Leydig cell: regulation and implications for paracrine control of Sertoli cell function. Endocrinology 122 (2): 749-55

Franchimont P, Croze F, Demoulin A, Bologne R, Hustin J (1981) Effect of inhibin on rat testicular desoxyribonculeic acid (DNA) synthesis in vitro. Acta Endocrinol (Copenh) 98: 312-320

Gerendai I, Shaha C, Gunsalus G, Bardin CW (1986) The effects of opioid receptor antagonists suggest that testicular opiates reduglate Sertoli and Leydig cell function in the neonatal rat. Endocrinology 118: 2039-2044

Gizang-Ginsberg E, Wolgemuth DJ (1985) Localization of mRANs in the mouse testes by in situ hybridization: distribution of alpha- tubulin and developmental stage specificity of pro- opiomelanocortin transcripts. Dev Biol 111: 293-305

Gizang-Ginsberg E, Wolgemuth DJ (1987) Expression of the proopiomelanocortin gene is developmentally regulated and affected by germ cells in the male mouse reproductive system. Proc Natl Acad Sci USA 84 (6): 1600-1604

Grossman A (1983) Brain opiates and neuroendocrine function. Clin Endocrinol Metab 12: 725-746

Hedger MP, Drummond AE, Robertson DM, Risbridger GP, de Kretser DM (1989) Inhibin and activin regulate (3H) thymidine uptake by rat thymocytes and 3T3 cells in vitro. Mol Cell Endocrinol 61: 133-138

Howlett TA, Rees LH (1987) Endogenous opioid peptides and human reproduction. Oxf Rev Reprod Biol 9: 260-293

Juniewicz PE, Keeney DS, Ewing LL (1988) Effect of adrenocorticotropin and other proopiomelanocortin-derived peptides on testosterone secretion by the in vitro perfused testis. Endocrinology 122 (3): 891-898

Kew D, Kilpatrick DL (1989) Expression and regulation of the proenkephalin gene in rat Sertoli cells. Mol Endocrinol 3 (1): 179-184

Kilpatrick DL, Borland K, Jin DF (1987) Differential expression of opioid peptide genes by testicular germ cells and somatic cells. Proc Natl Acad Sci USA 84 (16): 5695-5699

Kilpatrick DL, Howells RD, Noe M, Bailey CL, Udenfriend S (1985) Expression of preproenkephalin-like mRNA and its peptide products in mammalian testis and ovary. Proc Natl Acad Sci USA 82: 7467- 7469

Kilpatrick DL, Milette CF (1986) Expression of proenkephalin messenger RNA by mouse spermatogenic cells. Proc Natl Acad Sci USA 83: 5015-5018

Kilpatrick DL, Rosenthal JL (1986) The proenkephalin gene is widely expressed within the male and female reproductive systems of the rat and hamster. Endocrinology 119 (1): 370-374

Krishnan KA, Sluss PM, Reichert LE Jr (1986) Low molecular weight FSH binding inhibitor in bovine testis. J Androl 7: 42-48

Lacaze-Masmonteil T, de Keyzer Y, Luton JP, Kahn A, Bertagna X (1987) Characterization of proopiomelanocortin transcripts in human nonpituitary tissues. Proc Natl Acad Sci USA 84 (20): 7261- 7265

Lebouille JL, Burbach JP, de Kloet ER, Rommerts FF (1986) γ-Endorphin-generating endopeptidase: distribution in body tissues and cellular localization in rat testis. Endocrinology 118 (1): 372-376

Margioris AN, Liotta AS, Vaudry H, Bardin CW, Kreiger DT (1983) Characterisation of proopiomelanocortin-related peptides in rat testes. Endocrinology 113: 663-671

Marshall GR, Jöckenhovel F, Lüdecke D, Nieschlag E (1986) Maintenance of complete but quantitatively reduced spermatogenesis in hypophysectomised monkeys by testosterone alone. Acta Endocrinol (Copenh) 113: 424-431

Marshall GR, Nieschlag E (1987) The role of FSH in male reproduction. In: Sheth AR (ed) Inhibins: isolation, estimation and physiology, vol 1. CRC, Boca Raton, pp 3-15

Matsumoto AM, Bremner WJ (1987) Endocrinology of the hypothalamic-pituitary-testicular axis with particular reference to the hormonal control of spermatogenesis. Ballieres Clin Endocrinol Metab 1: 71-87

McMurray CT, Devi L, Calavetta L, Douglass JO (1989) Regulated expression of the prodynorphin gene in the R2C Leydig tumour cell line. Endocrinology 124: 49-59

Meites J, Bruni JF, van Vugt DA, Smith AF (1979) Relation of endogenous opioid peptides and morphine to neuroendocrine function. Life Sci 24: 1235-1336

Melner MH, Puett D (1984) Evidence for the synthesis of multiple pro-opiomelanocortin-like precursors in murine Leydig tumor cells. Arch Biochem Biophys 232 (1): 197-201

Morley JE (1981) The endocrinology of the opiates and opioid peptides. Metabolism 30: 195-207

Morris PL, Vale WW, Bardin CW (1987) β-endorphin regulation of FSH-stimulated inhibin production is a component of a short loop system in testis. Biochem Biophys Res Commun 148 (3): 1513- 1519

Nieschlag E, Bartlett JMS (1989) Testes. In: Bettendorf G, Breckwoldt M (eds) Reproduktionsmedizin. Fischer Stuttgart, pp 100-111

Orth J (1986) FSH-induced Sertoli cell proliferation in the developing rat is modified by β-endorphin production in the testis. Endocrinology 119: 1876-1878

Parvinen M (1982) Regulation of the seminiferous epithelium. endocr Rev 3: 404-417

Saint-Pol P, Peyrat PJ, Engelhardt RP, Leroy-Martin B (1986) Immunohistochemical localization of enkephalins in adult rat testis. Evidence of a gonadotrophin control. Andrologia 18: 485- 488

Saint-Pol P, Herman E, Tramu G (1988) Paracrine factors in adult rat testis. Gonadotrophin control of opioids and LHRH like peptide. Andrologia 20: 173-181

Schulze W, Davidoff MS, Holstein AF, Schirren C (1987) Processing of testicular biopsies fixed in Stieve's solution for visualization of substance P-and methionine-enkephalin-like immunoreactivity in Leydig cells. Andrologia 19 (4): 419-422

Setchell BP (1980) The functional significance of the blood–testis barrier. J Androl 1: 3-10

Shaha C, Liotta SA, Kreiger DT, Bardin CW (1984) The ontogeny of immunreactive-β-endorphin in fetal, neonatal, and pubertal testes from mouse and hamster. Endocrinology 114: 1584-1591

Sharpe RM (1982) The hormonal regulation of the Leydig cell. Oxf Rev Reprod Biol 4: 241-317

Sharpe RM (1984) Bibliography with review on intragonadal hormones. Bibliogr Reprod 44: C1-C26

Sharpe RM (1986) Paracrine control of the testis. Clin Endocrinol Metab 15: 185-207

Sharpe RM, Cooper I (1987) Comparison of the effects on purified leydig cells of four hormones (oscytocin, vasopression, opiates and LHRH) with suggested paracrine roles in the testis. J Ends 113: 89-96

Skinner MK, Fritz IB (1985a) Testicular peritubular cells secreted a protein under androgen control that modulates Sertoli cell function (rat). Proc Natl Acad Sci USA 82: 114-118

Skinner MK, Fritz IB (1985b) Androgen stimulation of Sertoli cell function is enhanced by peritubular cells. Mol Cell Endocrinol 40: 115-122

Skinner MK (1989) Peritubular myoid cell-Sertoli cell interactions which regulate testis function and growth. In: Serio M (ed) Perspectives in andrology. Raven, New York, pp 175-182 (Serono symposia, vol 53)

Srinath BV, Wickings EJ, Witting C, Nieschlag E (1983) Active immunisation with follicle stimulating hormone for fertility control: a 4 ½ year study in male rhesus monkeys. Fertil Steril 40: 110-117

Tsong SD, Phillips D, Halmi N, Liotta AS, Mariioris A, Bardin CW, Krieger DT (1982) ACTH and β-endorphin-related peptides are present in multiple sites in the reproductive tract in the male rat. Endocrinology 110: 2204-2206

Tsonis CG, Sharpe RM (1986) Dual gonadal control of follicle stimulating hormone. Nature 321: 724-725

Unni E, Rao MRS (1986) Androgen binding protein levels and FSH binding to testicular membranes in vitamin A deficient rats and during subsequent replenishment with vitamin A. J Steroid Biochem 25: 579-583

Van Dissel-Emiliani FMF, Grootenhuis AJ, de Jong FH, de Rooij DG (1988) Local action of inhibin in the testis (Abstr 1912). In: Proceedings of the Vth European Workshop on molecular and cellular endocrinology of the testis

Verhoeven G, Cailleau J (1988) Follicle-stimulating hormone and androgens increase the concentration of the androgen receptor in Sertoli cells. Endocrinology 122: 1541-1550

Wickings EJ, Usadel KH, Dathe G, Nieschlag E (1980) The role of follicle stimulating hormone in testicular function of the mature rhesus monkey. Acta Endocrinol (Copenh) 95: 117-128

Yoshikawa K, Aizawa T (1988a) Enkephalin precursor gene expression in postmeiotic germ cells. Biochem Biophys Res Commun 151 (2): 664-671

Yoshikawa K, Aizawa T (1988b) Expression of the enkephalin precursor gene in rat Sertoli cells. Regulation by follicle- stimulating hormone. FEBS Lett 237 (1-2): 183-186

Yoshikawa K, Aizawa T, Nozawa A (1989a) Phorbol ester regulates the abundance of enkephalin precursor mRNA but not of amyloid β-protein precursor mRNA in rat testicular peritubular cells. Biochem Biophys Res Commun 161 (2): 568-575

Yoshikawa K, Maruyama K, Aizawa T, Yamamoto A (1989b) A new species of enkephalin precursor mRNA with a distinct 5'- untranslated region in haploid germ cells. FEBS Lett 246 (1-2): 193-196

Role of β-Endorphin in the Ovary: In Vitro Studies of Porcine Ovaries and Individual Follicles[*]

G. WESTHOF, J. BENSCH, and W.L. BRAENDLE

Introduction

Evidence for a local ovarian production of β-endorphin has been reported for several species, e.g., sheep, mouse, rat, and human (Lim et al. 1983; Shaha et al. 1984; Aleem et al. 1986; Adams and Cicero 1989). Concentrations of β-endorphin in ovarian follicular fluid were reported to be significantly higher than in peripheral blood, suggesting a local ovarian secretion (Petraglia et al. 1985; Aleem et al. 1987). Recently, a periovulatory increase of β-endorphin was found in women with a normal cycle. Oral contraceptives abolished this mid-cycle increase, suggesting an ovarian contribution to the peripheral pool of β-endorphin (Comitini et al. 1989).

A reasonable hypothesis for the role of β-endorphin in the reproductive system has been established only for the testis (Fabbri et al. 1989): that in the male, β-endorphin may be a key factor inhibiting reproductive functions in stressful situations, when a rise in corticotropin-releasing factor (CRF) secretion occurs. CRF could be the nodal peptide which stimulates β-endorphin production. Inhibition via β-endorphin may then act at three levels: in the brain (sexual behavior), in the pituitary (inhibition of LH secretion), and in the testis (inhibition of tubular function). In the female, however, the local (or general) function of β-endorphin in the gonads seems far from being elucidated.

For our in vitro study on β-endorphin in the ovary, the pig was selected as a model because ample numbers of fresh porcine ovaries in different stages of the estrous cycle were readily available at a local abattoir. By immunohistochemical methods we sought to determine the ovarian structures which produce β-endorphin. Using an in vitro follicle incubation system, we sought to characterize the type of follicle which secretes the principle amount of β-endorphin and to compare the β-endorphin secretion of viable follicles to that of atretic follicles of similar size. Inspired by the finding that β-endorphin concentrations in follicular fluid from patients with polycystic ovaries were higher than those in follicular fluid from normal women (Aleem et al. 1987), we hypothesized that β-endorphin could be an atresia-inducing agent. Therefore, intact follicles were exposed to different media concentrations of β-endorphin in vitro and their morphology and steroid secretion pattern then examined.

* Supported by Deutsche Forschungsgemeinschaft grant Ho 388/6-1.

Materials and Methods

Immunohistochemistry

Fresh porcine ovaries in different stages of the estrous cycle were fixed for 48 h in Bouin's solution, sectioned, and embedded in paraffin. Sections were incubated with the primary β-endorphin antibody (radioimmunoassay grade, Incstar Corp., Stillwater, Maine, USA) for 16 h at 4°C. The primary antibody was raised in rabbits and directed against human β-endorphin. For staining of the sections, the avidin-biotin-peroxidase technique (Vectastain kit) was used. Preabsorption of the primary antibody by human β-endorphin (Sigma Chemicals, 5 μg/ml, 24h, 4°C) was used as control of the specificity of staining.

Follicle Incubation

Medium-sized follicles were separately dissected from preovulatory, porcine ovaries and incubated in 1 ml Medium 199 for 4 h. The desk-top incubator was placed on a rocker and connected to a gas inflow system (37°C, 5% CO_2, 95% O_2). Immediately after incubation, conditioned media were collected and follicles separately fixed in Bouin's solution. Media were frozen at −20°C until assayed for hormone concentrations. Incubated follicles were histologically classified as *viable* if all granulosa cell layers were intact. Follicles which demonstrated disintegrated and pyknotic granulosa cells were classified as *atretic*.

Steroid and Protein Assays

Media concentrations of estradiol (E_2), testosterone (T), androstenedione (A), and progesterone (P) were determined by established radioimmunoassays as previously described in detail (Westhof et al. 1989). Radioimmunoassay kits for β-endorphin and adrenocorticotropin (ACTH) were from Incstar Corp. and from Diagnostic Products Corporation (Hermann Biermann GmbH, Diagnostica, Bad Nauheim, FRG), respectively.

Results

Immunohistochemical Localization of β-Endorphin

Viable follicles demonstrated an intensely stained stratum granulosum. Staining of the theca interna was less intense. A typical section from a tertiary, viable follicle is shown in Fig. 1. Control sections (preabsorption of primary antibody with human β-endorphin) did not show any significant staining. In atretic follicles, the theca interna was stained more intensely than in viable follicles. Figure 2 depicts an example of a late atretic follicle; all granulosa cell layers were disintegrated and pyknotic. Significant staining was also seen in corpora

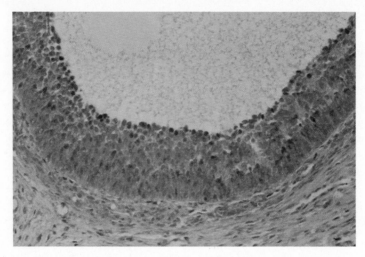

Fig. 1. Immunohistochemical localization of β-endorphin: typical section of viable, tertiary follicle

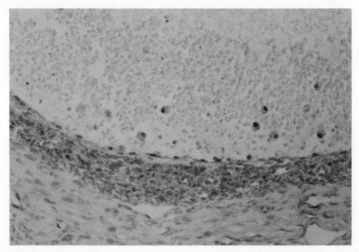

Fig. 2. Immunohistochemical localization of β-endorphin: typical section of (late) atretic, tertiary follicle

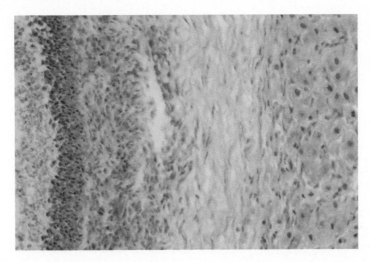

Fig. 3. Immunohistochemical localization of β-endorphin: typically stained corpus luteum neighbouring a viable follicle

lutea, but this was less intense than that in granulosa cells from viable follicles. Figure 3 shows a typically stained corpus luteum neighboring a viable follicle. The interstitial tissue remained unstained.

Gonadotropin Stimulation of Steroidal Secretion

To validate the incubation system, we first demonstrated a stimulatory effect of follicle stimulating hormone (FSH) and luteinizing hormone (LH) on follicular steroidal secretion in vitro. When exposed to 1 μg or 10 μg highly purified porcine FSH, viable follicles significantly increased their secretion of E_2, T, A, and P (Fig. 4). Viable follicles secreted more E_2 than T, before and during FSH exposure. In contrast, atretic follicles typically secreted less E_2 than T. In addition, the amount of E_2 secreted was inversely related to the progress of atresia (not shown). Furthermore, highly purified porcine LH increased follicular secretion of E_2, T, A and P in a dose-dependent manner (Fig.5). These data obtained from FSH and LH stimulations indicate that the follicles remained functionally intact when incubated in vitro. The follicle incubation system was therefore considered an adequate method to evaluate the secretion of β-endorphin by viable and atretic follicles and the response of β-endorphin secretion to gonadotropin stimulation in vitro.

Secretion of β-Endorphin and ACTH In Vitro

Concentrations of β-endorphin in incubation media from individual follicles were in the pmol/l range (Fig. 6). Viable and atretic follicles secreted similar

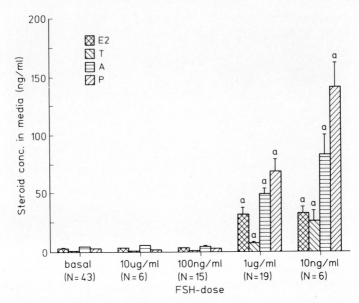

Fig. 4. Incubation of medium-sized, viable follicles in vitro for 4 h: FSH stimulation of steroid secretion. *a*, $p < 0.001$ (vs. basal)

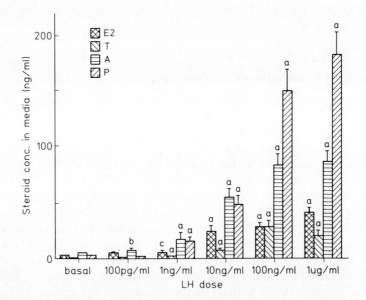

Fig. 5. Incubation of medium-sized, viable follicles in vitro for 4 h: LH stimulation of steroid secretion. *a*, $p < 0.001$; *b*, $p < 0.01$; *c*, $p < 0.05$ (vs. basal)

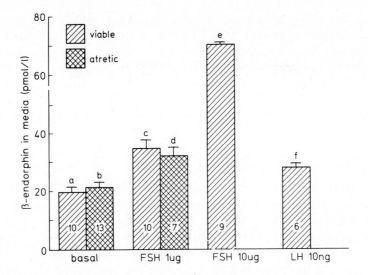

Fig. 6. Secretion of β-endorphin by viable and atretic follicles incubated for 4 h in vitro. Significant differences (p) between groups (U test): a < c < e; b < d

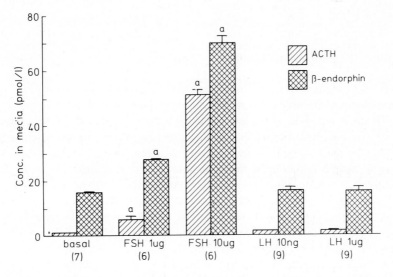

Fig. 7. Secretion β-endorphin and ACTH by viable follicles incubated for 4 h in vitro. a, p < 0.001 (vs. basal)

amounts of β-endorphin, under basal conditions as well as under exposure to 1 μg FSH. β-Endorphin secretion by viable follicles was increased by FSH in a dose-dependent manner. To provide further evidence that the substance we measured in incubation media was actually β-endorphin, ACTH was determined as well. A new set of the same type of experiment (Fig. 7) had to be established to ensure that media had not been thawed prior to ACTH measurements. All data shown in Fig. 7 were obtained from viable follicles. Again, FSH enhanced the secretion of β-endorphin in a dose-dependent manner, whereas LH had no effect. The quantity of ACTH secreted by the same follicles was smaller than that of β-endorphin, but the response pattern to FSH was similar to that of β-endorphin. Also ACTH did not show any response to LH when compared to controls.

In Vitro Exposure of Follicles to β-Endorphin

When viable follicles were exposed to β-endorphin in concentrations ranging from 100 pg to 1 μg, no significant alteration of the steroid secretion pattern was observed after 4 h incubation. Combined treatments of follicles with β-endorphin and FSH or LH did not significantly alter the steroid secretion either, in comparison to follicles treated with FSH or LH alone. The incidence of atresia among β-endorphin-treated follicles was not significantly different from controls in vivo and in vitro or from gonadotropin-exposed follicles. Neither did combinations of β-endorphin and gonadotropins affect follicular morphology.

Discussion and Conclusions

The results obtained from immunohistochemical determinations of β-endorphin in porcine ovaries indicate that this opioid peptide is produced in the cyclic ovarian structures, i.e., in preantral and antral follicles and in corpora lutea. In viable follicles, both granulosa and theca cells seem to produce β-endorphin; granulosa cells, however, seem to be the principle source. In atretic follicles, the theca interna seems to be the main source of production.

Individual porcine follicles of medium size which were studied in an in vitro incubation system remained morphologically and functionally intact. The experimental procedure did not affect their histological appearance, and follicular steroid secretion in vitro could be enhanced by adding FSH or LH to incubation media. In this system, viable and atretic follicles secreted similar amounts of β-endorphin, indicating that atretic follicles are not only important sources of steroids but also seem to contribute significantly to ovarian secretion of opioid peptides. When data from immunohistochemistry and in vitro incubations are taken together, the theca interna seems to enhance its production and secretion of β-endorphin once the follicle becomes atretic, thereby "compensating" the lack of granulosal β-endorphin production.

FSH but not LH stimulated the secretion of β-endorphin. Although a relatively high dose of FSH was required to demonstrate this stimulatory effect, an LH contamination does not account for the β-endorphin increase in media: both preparations of porcine gonadotropins were highly purified. Since another proopiomelanocortin (POMC) derivative, ACTH, was secreted simultaneously by the same follicles and did similarly respond to FSH but not LH, the immunoreactivity found in follicle incubation media was very likely due to β-endorphin, rather than a nonspecific phenomenon. Therefore, our data indicate that the porcine ovary produces and secretes β-endorphin and other POMC derivatives which are regulated by FSH. However, their local biological role still remains to be determined. A longer time of in vitro exposure of follicles to β-endorphin might be required to demonstrate alterations of follicular steroido-genesis and morphology. Alternatively, β-endorphin secreted by the ovary could lack a local role but could take part in the endocrine communication system between ovary and pituitary or hypothalamus, as shown for inhibin or steroids.

References

Adams ML, Cicero TJ (1989) The ontogeny of immunoreactive β-endorphin and β-lipotropin in the rat ovary. Biochem Biophys Res Commun 159: 1171-1176

Aleem FA, Omar RA, El Tabbakh GH (1986) Immunoreactive β- endorphin in human ovaries. Fertil Steril 45: 507-511

Aleem FA, El Tabbak GH, Omar RA, Southren AL (1987) Ovarian follicular fluid β-endorphin levels in normal and polycystic ovaries. Am J Obstet Gynecol 156: 1197-1200

Comitini G, Petraglia F, Facchinetti F, Monaco M, Volpe A, Genazzani AR (1989) Effect of oral contraceptives or dexamethasone on plasma β-endorphin during the menstrual cycle. Fertil Steril 51: 46-50

Fabbri A, Jannini EA, Gnessi L, Ulisse S, Moretti C, Isidori A (1989) Neuroendocrine control of male reproductive function. The opioid system as a model of control at multiple sites. J Steroid Biochem 32: 145-150

Lim AT, Lolait S, Barlow JW, Wai Sum O, Zois I, Toh BH, Funder JW (1983) Immunoreactive β-endorphin in sheep ovary. Nature 303: 709-711

Petraglia F, Segre A, Facchinetti F, Campanini D, Ruspa M, Genazzani AR (1985) β-endorphin and met-enkephalin in peritoneal and ovarian fluids of fertile and postmenopausal women. Fertil Steril 44: 615

Shaha C, Margioris A, Liotta AS, Krieger DT, Bardin CW (1984) Demonstration of immunoreactive β-endorphin-and gamma3-melano-cyte-stimulating hormone-related peptides in the ovaries of neonatal, cyclic, and pregnant mice. Endocrinology 115: 378-384

Westhof G, Westhof KF, Ahmad N, di Zerega GS (1989) Alteration of follicular steroid secretion and thecal morphology after in vitro exposure of individual pig follicles to follicle regulatory protein. J Reprod Fertil 87: 133-140

Human Plasma β-Endorphin Levels in Pregnant Women and in Newborns

W. DISTLER

Pregnancy, labor and delivery are potentially stressful states for the mother and fetus. Therefore, various researchers have measured β-endorphin in the peripheral plasma of women (a) during pregnancy, in labor, and after delivery; (b) in labor without and with epidural anesthesia; and (c) prior to and after induction of general or regional anesthesia for cesarian section. There have been also determinations of β-endorphin in the umbilical arterial and venous blood of newborns following spontaneous or operative vaginal and abdominal delivery, without and with fetal distress. It is the objective of this paper to summarize the data of other groups and to discuss our own measurements of maternal and neonatal β-endorphin in the light of other publications.

Radioimmunoassay for β-Endorphin

Plasma β-endorphin was measured with slight modifications according to the method of Shaaban et al. (1982). Briefly, 5 – 10 ml aliquots of plasma were extracted with silicic acid according to the method of Krieger et al. (1977), after approximately 2000 cpm ^{125}I-labeled β-endorphin had been added as recovery standard. The peptides were eluted with 0.1 N hydrochloric acid: acetone (3: 2, v: v) from the silicic acid precipitate, and the eluates were evaporated under a stream of dry air. The redissolved eluates were subjected to chromatography on a 180 × 6 mm Sephadex G-50 column to separate the β-endorphin fraction from β-lipotropin and other peptides as described by Shaaban et al. (1982).

The radioimmunoassay was performed as double-antibody method. The β-endorphin antiserum (Dr. Goebelsmann, Los Angeles, USA) did not exhibit any crossreaction with human α-MSH, human ACTH (1-39), methionine enkephalin, or leucine enkephalin. However, the antiserum crossreacted 33 % on a weight basis and 100 % on a molar basis with β-lipotropin. As second antibody we used a sheep anti-rabbit γ-globulin, and after further incubation for 3 h we added 15 % polyethylene glycol in phosphate-buffered saline to separate bound and unbound ^{125}I-labeled β-endorphin. The contents of the radioimmunoassay tubes were mixed and thereafter tubes were centrifuged at 4°C and 1.800g for 20 min. The supernatants were decanted and the pellets were subjected to γ-counting. If 5 ml of plasma were extracted the assay sensitivity was 10 pg/ml. The intra- and interassay coefficients of variation were 8 % and 13 %, respectively.

Maternal Plasma β-Endorphin Levels During Pregnancy, in Labor, and After Delivery

Plasma β-endorphin levels were lower in pregnant women than in nonpregnant controls (Table 1). During the second trimester β-endorphin concentrations showed a significant nadir. During early and advanced labor mean maternal plasma β-endorphin levels rose drastically and remained significantly elevated during the early postpartum period. The β-endorphin values measured by us in nonpregnant, pregnant, and parturient women were higher than those of Csontos et al. (1979), Wardlaw et al. (1979), and Goland et al. (1981), lower than those obtained by Wilkes et al. (1980), and agree with the data reported by Hoffman et al. (1984). As already mentioned, we found a significant decrease of plasma β-endorphin concentrations during the second trimester of pregnancy and our results are in agreement with Goebelsmann et al. (1984). However, Goland et al. (1981) observed marginally but not significantly higher β- endorphin levels in pregnant women. Genazzani et al. (1981) reported a significant decrease of maternal plasma β-endorphin between the 9th and 12th week of gestation and an increase near term as compared to nonpregnant women. Nevertheless, from our own findings and these of Goebelsmann et al. (1984), we conclude that in the absence of specific stressful stimuli, maternal plasma β-endorphin levels are decreased rather than increased throughtout pregnancy until labor begins.

With the onset of labor, maternal plasma β-endorphin concentrations rise and continue to be elevated during the early postpartum period. This is most consistent with the increase in ACTH secretion which has been reported to occur during labor and to peak at delivery (Allen et al. 1973). For this reason one

Table 1. Plasma β-endorphin concentrations (pg/ml) in nonpregnant controls and women during pregnancy and labor or 30 - 60 min post partum

	Mean	± S E	n
Nonpregnant controls	65	10.5	25
First trimester	50	5.6	15
Second trimester	29	2.3*	15
Third trimester	51	7.3	25
Early labor	187	35.6	12
Advanced labor	410	81.2	10
30-60 Min postpartum	156	25.1	15

* Significant difference from 1st and 3rd trimesters, Student's t test.

would expect to observe higher β-endorphin levels during advanced than during early labor. We found mean maternal plasma β-endorphin levels higher during late than during early labor, but the difference was not statistically significant (Table 1). However, Goland et al. (1981) measured significantly higher maternal β-endorphin concentrations in advanced first-stage labor, while Rust et al. (1980) found no significant difference between early and late labor maternal plasma β-endorphin concentrations. The observation that maternal plasma β-endorphin levels remain elevated for 30–60 min after delivery, considering the short half-life of β-endorphin (Reid et al. 1981), indicates that the maternal pituitary continues to secrete increased amounts of β-endorphin following the delivery (Goebelsmann et al. 1984).

Response of Maternal Plasma β-Endorphin Levels to Epidural Anesthesia in Active Labor

According to the data of Abboud et al. (1983b), mean plasma β-endorphin levels fell significantly in women during labor within 30–40 min following placement of an epidural catheter and activation with 0.5% bupivacaine or 2% 2-chloroprocaine. In controls who also were in active labor and received epidural catheter placement but saline instead of an anesthetic, mean plasma β-endorphin concentrations did not change significantly (Table 2). The observation that epidural anesthesia causes a decline in maternal plasma β-endorphin levels while uterine contractions and progress in labor continue, indicates that pain and/or pain-associated stress are major stimuli of pituitary β-endorphin release rather than labor per se (Goebelsmann et al. 1984). These findings are in agreement with those of Thomas et al. (1982), who was able to demonstrate that extradural blocks applied to women in active labor resulted in decreased peripheral plasma β-endorphin concentrations.

Table 2. Plasma β-endorphin concentrations (pg/ml) in women in active labor prior to and 30-40 min after induction of epidural anesthesia, as compared to controls who underwent epidural catheter placement but received saline instead of anesthetic. (Goebelsmann et al. 1984)

	Active epidural anesthesia group ($n = 15$)		Epidural catheter control group ($n = 10$)	
	Mean	± S E	Mean	± S E
Before	189	32	223	71
After	98	12	193	47
p[a]	< 0.02		N S	

[a] Student's t test.

Maternal Plasma β-Endorphin Levels After Induction of General or Regional Anesthesia

In 14 patients who underwent general anesthesia for cesarean section, mean plasma β-endorphin levels increased significantly (Abboud et al. 1983a). However, mean plasma β-endorphin concentrations of patients who received regional anesthesia did not rise significantly after induction of regional anesthesia (Table 3). These findings of Abboud et al. (1983a) are consistent with the data of Pflug and Halter (1981), who observed that plasma epinephrine, norepinephrine, growth hormone, and cortisol concentrations are elevated in patients undergoing general but not regional anesthesia. While a more detailed consideration of the many aspects and clinical implications of these interesting data is beyond the scope of this paper, it appears possible to conclude that induction of regional anesthesia is less stressful than general anesthesia for women undergoing cesarean section (Goebelsmann et al. 1984).

Table 3. Plasma β-endorphin concentrations (pg/ml) in patients prior to and following induction of general endotracheal or regional anesthesia.(Goebelsmann et al. 1984)

	General anesthesia ($n = 14$)		Regional anesthesia ($n = 26$)	
	Mean	± S E	Mean	± S E
Before	159	25.6	154	17.7
After	387	30.8	165	16.6
p^a	< 0.025		N S	

[a] Student's *t* test.

Determinations of Plasma β-Endorphin Concentrations in the Umbilical Cord Blood of Newborns

Shaaban et al. (1982) studied human β-endorphin concentrations in umbilical cord blood obtained from newborn infants delivered by various routes and modes with and without apparent intrapartum fetal distress. It could be demonstrated that the mean umbilical venous β-endorphin concentrations measured after normal spontaneous vaginal delivery without fetal distress did not differ from those found after elective cesarean section, emergency cesarean section, or delivery by forceps or vacuum in the absence of fetal distress (Fig. 1). However, in conjunction with fetal distress, umbilical venous β-endorphin levels were significantly higher both after forceps or vacuum delivery and after emergency cesarean section.

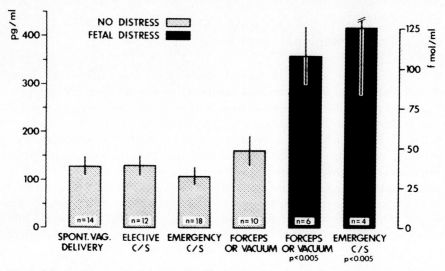

Fig. 1. β-Endorphin concentrations in umbilical venous plasma obtained from newborn infants delivered by various routes and modes with and without apparent intrapartum fetal distress. Bars represent means ±SE (Shaaban et al. 1982)

This last study indicates that neither the presence or absence of labor nor the route or mode of delivery affect the umbilical venous plasma β-endorphin concentrations, but in response to fetal distress β-endorphin levels rise promptly and significantly. This is in agreement with data of Wardlaw et al. (1979), who demonstrated a significant inverse correlation between umbilical plasma β-endorphin concentrations and arterial pO_2 and pH values, suggesting that fetal hypoxia and/or acidosis are related to β-endorphin release.

In contradistinction to the study of Wardlaw et al. (1979), Shaaban et al. (1982) demonstrated that umbilical venous plasma β-endorphin concentrations are higher than umbilical arterial plasma β-endorphin levels in the absence of fetal distress. Recent findings of Fraioli and Genazzani (1980) or Liotta and Krieger (1980) are in agreement with the latter data, suggesting that the placenta contributes to the pool of circulating fetal β-endorphin.

However, Goebelsmann et al. (1984) reported that in the presence of fetal distress umbilical arterial β-endorphin concentrations appear to rise more extensively than umbilical venous β-endorphin levels. This observation is consistent with the findings of Facchinetti et al. (1982) that β-endorphin is present in the plasma of newborns during the first 24 h of life. Considering the short half life of β-endorphin the data seem to indicate that at term the fetal pituitary is capable of releasing β-endorphin in response to stress.

In order to elucidate the role of endorphins at birth and in the early neonatal period Pohjavuori et al. (1985) measured plasma immunoreactive β-endorphin and cortisol levels in newborns during the first 2 h of life after elective cesarean section and after spontaneous vaginal delivery. As shown in Table 4, at the age of 2 h the mean plasma concentrations of β-endorphin were higher after cesarean

Table 4. Plasma concentrations of immunoreactive β-endorphin and cortisol in maternal and cord blood after elective cesarean section and after spontaneous labor. Means ± SE. (Pohjavuori et al. 1985)

	Elective cesarean section ($n = 10$)	Spontaneous labor ($n = 17$)
β-Endorphin (ng/ml)		
Maternal plasma	49 ± 8.2 **	594 ± 98
Cord venous plasma	111 ± 24	181 ± 29
Newborn venous plasma at age 2 h	117 ± 21 *	64 ± 7
Cortisol (nmol/l)		
Maternal plasma	1032 ± 74 **	2041 ± 102
Cord arterial plasma	327 ± 53 **	818 ± 83
Cord venous plasma	327 ± 27 **	735 ± 78
Newborn venous plasma at age 2 h	705 ± 90	659 ± 43

Comparisons between groups $*p < 0.005$, $**p < 0.001$.

Table 5. Umbilical venous plasma β-endorphin concentrations in mature and premature newborns after vaginal delivery and cesarean section

	Mature infants β-endorphin (pg/ml)			Premature infants β-endorphin (pg/ml)		
	Mean	± S E	n	Mean	± S E	n
Vaginal delivery	115	25.6	15	353	65.3	7
Cesarean section	131	21.2	15	240	36.4	14

section than after spontaneous labor. These results show that, irrespective of the route and mode, delivery is stressful to the newborn infant. In newborns delivered by cesarean section, the stress response seems to come about 2 h after birth. The sustained β-endorphin secretion in newborn infants after elective cesarean section may have clinical significance, since the role of endorphins in respiratory difficulties should be taken into account (Chernick 1981).

Recently we compared umbilical venous plasma β-endorphin concentrations in premature and mature newborn infants after vaginal delivery or elective cesarean section (Distler et al. 1988). Our data indicate that in the premature infants the β-endorphin levels after vaginal and abdominal delivery were significantly higher than in mature newborns (Table 5). It appears quite conceivable that for premature infants delivery is more stressful and therefore most likely the release of β-endorphin from the fetal pituitary is more pronounced. Since high opioid levels can cause respiratory and circulatory difficulties, premature infants are more exposed to risk of these problems (Davidson et al. 1987; Orlowski et al. 1982).

The physiological role of β-endorphin in the fetoplacental unit and newborn infant remains incompletely understood, although it may be assumed that β-endorphin and perhaps other neurotransmitters modulate the central regulation of hypoxia-induced changes in fetal heart rate patterns (Shaaban et al. 1982). Goodlin (1981) was able to normalize the severely suppressed beat-to-beat variability of the heart rate of an acidotic fetus by administrating the narcotic antagonist naloxone to the mother, while the fetal acidosis remained essentially unchanged. There is also a good possibility that part of the physiological role of β-endorphin is to reduce the pain the fetus must suffer during delivery (Lord et al. 1976). However, neither the presence or absence of uterine contractions nor the route or mode of delivery affects umbilical venous plasma concentrations of β-endorphin (Goebelsmann et al. 1984). While maternal general analgesia has no apparent effect upon umbilical cord plasma β-endorphin levels, maternal plasma β-endorphin decreases significantly in response to epidural anesthesia during labor (Abboud et al. 1983b). Furthermore, it could be demonstrated that maternal plasma β-endorphin levels rise during active labor up to the time of delivery, suggesting that labor pain is a likely stimulus for maternal circulating β-endorphin levels, in contradistinction to β-endorphin concentrations in the fetoplacental circulation, which appear to respond primarily to hypoxia (Shaaban et al. 1982). Anyway, the data are consistent with the hypothesis that peripheral plasma β-endorphin concentrations reflect stress in both mother and fetus.

References

Abboud TK, Noueihed R, Khoo SS, Hoffman DI, Varakian L, Henriksen E Goebelsmann U (1983a) Effects of induction of general and regional anesthesia for cesarean section on maternal plasma β-endorphin levels. Am J Obstet Gynecol 146: 927-930

Abboud TK, Sarkis F, Hung II, Khoo SS, Varakian L, Henriksen E, Noueihed R, Goebelsmann U (1983b) Effects of epidural anesthesia during labor on maternal plasma beta beta-endorphin levels. Anesthesiology 59: 1-5

Allen JP, Coor DM, Kendall JW, McGilvra R (1973) Maternal-fetal ACTH relationship in man. J Clin Endocrinol Metab 37: 230-234

Chernick V (1981) Endorphins and ventilatory control. N Engl J Med 304: 1227-1228

Csontos K, Rust M, Höllt V, Mahr W, Kromer W, Teschemacher HJ (1979) Elevated plasma β-endorphin levels in pregnant women and their neonates. Life Sci 25: 835-844

Davidson S, Gil-Ad I, Rogovin H, Laron Z, Reisner SH (1987) Cardiorespiratory depression and plasma β-endorphin levels in low-birth-weight infants during the first day of life. Am J Dis Child 41: 145-148

Distler W, Schwenzer T, Umbach G, Graf M (1988) β-Endorphin bei Frühgeburten und reifen Neugeborenen nach vaginaler und abdominaler Entbindung. Geburtshilfe Frauenheilkd 48: 140-142

Facchinetti F, Bagnoli F, Bracci R, Genazzani AR (1982) Plasma opioids in the first hours of life. Pediat Res 16: 95-98

Fraioli F, Genazzani AR (1980) Human placental β-endorphin. Gynecol Obstet Invest 11: 37-44

Genazzani AR, Facchinetti I, Parrini D (1981) β-Lipotropin and β-endorphin plasma levels during pregnancy. Clin Endocrinol (Oxf) 14: 409-418

Goebelsmann U, Abboud TK, Hoffman DI, Hung TT (1984) Beta- endorphin in pregnancy. Eur J Obstet Gynecol Reprod Biol 17: 77-89

Goland RS, Wardlaw SL, Stark RI, Frantz AG (1981) Human plasma β-endorphin during pregnancy, labor and delivery. J Clin Endocrinol Metab 52: 74-78

Goodlin RC (1981) Naloxone and its possible relationship to fetal endorphin levels and fetal distress. Am J Obstet Gynecol 139: 16-19

Hoffman DI, Abboud TK, Haase HR, Hung TT, Goebelsmann U (1984) Plasma β-endorphin concentrations prior to and during pregnancy, in labor and after delivery. Am J Obstet Gynecol 150: 492-498

Krieger DT, Liotta AS, Li CH (1977) Human plasma immunoreactive β-lipotropin: correlation with basal and stimulated plasma ACTH concentration. Life Sci 21: 1771-1777

Liotta AS Krieger DT (1980) In vitro biosynthesis and comparative translational processing of immunoreactive precursor corticotropin/β-endorphin by human placental and pituitary. cells. Endocrinology 106: 1504-1511

Lord JAH, Waterfield A, Hughes J, Kosterlitz HW (1976) Multiple opiate receptors. In: Kosterlitz HW (ed) Opiates and endogenous opioid peptides. North-Holland, Amsterdam p 275

Orlowski JP, Lonsdale D, Denko CW (1982) β-Endorphin levels in infant apnea syndrome: a preliminary communication. Cleve Clin Q 49: 87-92

Pflug AE, Halter JB (1981) Effect of spinal anesthesia on adrenergic tone and neuroendocrine response to surgical stress in humans. Anesthesiology 55: 120-126

Pohjavuori M, Rovamo L, Laatikainen T (1985) Plasma immunoreactive β-endorphin and cortisol in the newborn infant after elective caesarean section and after spontaneous labour. Eur J Obstet Gynecol Reprod Biol 19: 67-74

Reid RL, Hoff JD, Yen SSC, Li CH (1981) Effects of endogenous β-endorphin on pituitary hormone secretion and its disappearance rate in normal subjects. J Clin Endocrinol Metab 52: 1179-1184

Rust M, Csontos K, Mahr W, Höllt V, Zilker T, Hegemann M, Teschemacher H (1980) Zum Verhalten von β-Endorphin in der Perinatalperiode. Geburtshilfe Frauenheilkd 40:769-774

Shaaban MM, Hung TT, Hoffmann DI, Lobo RA, Goebelsmann U (1982) β-Endorphin and β-lipotropin concentration in umbilical cord blood. Am J Obstet Gynecol 144: 560-568

Thomas TA, Fletcher JE, Hill RG (1982) Influence of medication, pain and progress in labor on plasma β-endorphin like immunoreactivity. Br J Anaesth 54: 401-408

Wardlaw SL., Stark RI, Baxi L, Frantz AG (1979) Plasma β- endorphin and β-lipotropin in the human fetus at delivery: correlation with arterial pH and pO2. J Clin Endocrinol Metab 49: 888-891

Wilkes MM, Stewart RD, Bruni JF, Quigley ME, Yen SSC, Ling N, Chretien M (1980) A specific homologous radioimmunoassay for human β-endorphin: direct measurement in biological fluids. J Clin Endocrinol Metab 50: 309-315

Stress and Opioids

Opioid Peptides and Stress: The Sympathetic Nervous System and Pituitary-Adrenal Axis

A. GROSSMAN

Introduction

The families of endogenous opioid peptides (endorphins, enkephalins, and dynorphins) are distributed throughout the central nervous system, with both the peptides themselves and their putative receptors especially concentrated in nuclei concerned with neuroendocrine regulation, particularly the hypothalamus. Whatever their direct effects on gonadal function, opioid peptides can indirectly modulate reproductive fitness by regulating the output and fine-tuning of the principal mammalian stress axes, the sympatho-adrenomedullary system and the hypothalamo-pituitary-adrenal (H-P-A) axis. From a vast field, the current review will concentrate on some of our own work in order to obtain a potential overview of the regulation of these systems, with particular reference to the human. Full lists of references can be found in a number of reviews cited.

The Sympathetic Nervous System

While there are extensive and contradictory data on the role of opioid peptides in the control of the sympatho-adrenomedullary axis in the rat, evidence in the human is relatively slim. Drew et al. (1946) originally noted that morphine was a sympathodepressor, and this was essentially confirmed by the more detailed studies of Zelis et al. (1974) some 30 years later. We had been interested in the neuroendocrine profile of the long- acting met-enkephalin analogue, DAMME (FK33-824, Sandoz, Basel, Switzerland), and during studies of the opioid control of vasopressin it was noted that subjects became posturally hypotensive following infusion of the enkephalin (Grossman et al. 1980). Subsequent investigation of the catecholamine responses to DAMME infusion showed that both plasma noradrenaline and adrenaline, but not circulating dopamine, were inhibited under basal conditions (Grossman et al. 1982a). Similarly, Rubin (1984) found that the same analogue inhibited the reflex tachcardyia to baro-ceptor-mediated hypotension, indicating suppression of sympathetic activity. This suggested that exogenous opioids might be particularly effective at inhibit-ing sympathetic function when the system was activated, and we therefore proceeded to look at other situations where increased sympathetic function might be expected. Insulin-induced hypoglycaemia is one such stimulus, causing massive increases in circulating adrenaline (similar to those seen in the clinical situation of a myocardial infarction) and, to a lesser extent, noradrenaline. As previously found, DAMME caused a small but significant lowering of the basal levels of both catecholamines, but, most importantly, produced a potent suppression of the hypoglycaemia-induced release (Bouloux et al. 1985). Other clinical studies also demonstrated that the μ- opiate receptor agonist fentanyl inhibited the catecholamine response to anaesthesia. Thus, there is good pharmacological evidence for opitate suppression of the sympatho-adrenomedullary axis in the human.

However, in order to demonstrate an effect of *endogenous* opioids, we employed the tactic of investigating the changes induced by the specific opiate antagonist naloxone. Previous work (reviewed in Bouloux and Grossman 1989) had not clearly shown any effect of naloxone on cardiovascular or sympathoadrenal parameters, but only low doses were used, i.e., those required to block the effects of exogenous morphine in clinical situations (0.4-0.8 mg). As there is now evidence for non-μ opiate receptors, such as δ-receptors and κ-receptors, which are 10-20 times less sensitive to naloxone, we used doses of naloxone increased by this order of magnitude. With this experimental paradigm, it was found that, whereas naloxone had no effect on circulating catecholamines under basal conditions (Bouloux et al. 1985, 1986), the increase in plasma adrenaline induced by hypoglycaemia was enhanced by approximately 100%. A similar degree of enhancement was seen in the adrenaline responses to acute physical exercise (Grossman et al. 1984), isometric hand grip (Lam et al. 1986), and the cold pressor test (Bouloux et al. 1986). Circulating noradrenaline principally represents spill-over from sympathetic postganglionic nerve endings and is therefore only an indirect measure of sympathetic activity; nevertheless, plasma noradrenaline levels to intense stimuli are also enhanced by about 20%-30% (Grossman et al. 1984; Bouloux et al. 1985). These increases in plasma catecholamines do not appear to be secondary to changes in metabolism or distribution, as 8 mg naloxone had no effect on the half-life of adrenaline infused into normal subjects (Bouloux et al. 1989; Fig. 1).

In order to study the opiate receptor subtype in more detail, a detailed dose–response study was carried out in the dose range of 25-250 μg/kg naloxone, using the rise in plasma adrenaline during the cold pressor test as the end-point. It was found that only 100 μg/kg and above was able to significantly enhance the rise in adrenaline, suggesting that either δ- receptors or κ-receptors are involved in this process (Bouloux et al. 1989).

These studies therefore suggested that an endogenous opioid, probably acting at non-μ receptors, could modulate sympathoadrenal function during various forms of physical stress. However, the stressors used were not for the most part those that would be frequently met in normal life, and so it was decided to study a specifically mental stressor, the Stroop colour-word test. This protocol involved the administration of a totally automated, computer-generated mental

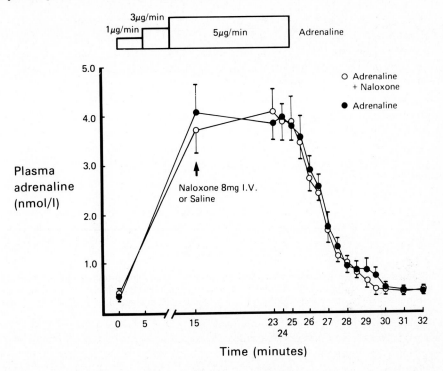

Fig. 1. Change in mean (± SE) plasma adrenaline following an infusion of adrenaline and then either 8 mg naloxone or an equal volume of saline, in eight normal subjects. Naloxone had no effect on the half-life of adrenaline. (From Bouloux et al. 1989)

stress test, with intermittent measurement of plasma catecholamines, blood pressure and pulse rate (Morris et al. 1990). While the elevations in catecholamines and blood pressure were relatively minor, the stress produced a significant rise in pulse rate in normal subjects which was markedly enhanced in the presence of a high dose (8 mg) of naloxone (Fig. 2). Thus, it would appear that any stimulus to the sympatho-adrenomedullary axis is accompanied by a parallel rise in endogenous opioid inhibition, which acts to damp down or attenuate sympathetic activity. McCubbin et al. (1985) demonstrated that individuals with a strong family history of hypertension may be relatively lacking in such tone, and the consequent cardiovascular lability may predispose to the later development of coronary heart disease. Our current studies involve an investigation of the effect of a continuous naloxone infusion on cardiovascular variables and plasma and urinary catecholamines in normal ambulant subjects, using ambulatory monitoring and recording, in order to identify the role of the opioids in normal physiology. Future work will need to identify the site of action

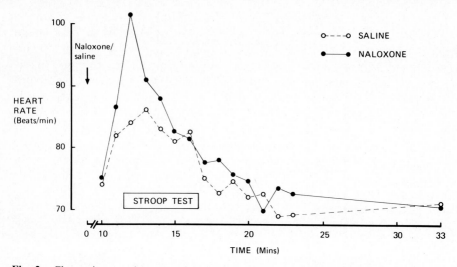

Fig. 2. Change in mean heart rate following mental stress (Stroop test) in the presence of either 8 mg naloxone or an equal volume of saline, in eight normal subjects. The rise in heart rate induced by the stress was significantly enhanced by opiate blockade with naloxone. (From Morris et al. 1990)

of these opioids (which is curently unknown in humans) and their significance in pathological states.

The Hypothalamo-Pituitary-Adrenal Axis

The inhibitory role of exogenous opioids on the H-P-A axis in humans is well established, using exogenous opiates such as morphine, methadone and nalorphine (McDonald et al. 1959; Delitala et al. 1983) and opiate peptides such as DAMME and β-endorphin (Gaillard et al. 1981; Allolio et al. 1982; Taylor et al. 1983). Conversely, naloxone causes an increase in basal H-P-A activity, leading to elevations in cortisol, adrenocorticotrophin (ACTH), and ACTH-related peptides (reviewed in Van Wimersma Greidanus and Grossman 1990). High doses of naloxone are required to both block opioid-induced suppression and elevate basal levels, similar to those needed to enhance stimulated adrenaline release (Grossman et al. 1986a; Bouloux et al. 1989). This tonic inhibition has a circadian variation, with minimal tone at night when activity in the H-P-A axis is lowest (Grossman et al. 1982b), and may be specifically antagonised by the α_1-adrenoceptor antagonist thymoxamine (Grossman and

Besser 1982). As the α_1-adrenoceptor control of the H-P-A occurs above the level of the pituitary (Al-Damluji et al. 1987), this suggests that the opioid modulation of ACTH occurs by regulation of the central control of corticotrophin releasing factors. However, the pituitary-adrenal response to exogenous corticotrophin releasing factor-41 (CRF-41) is attenuated by opioids such as DAMME (Allolio et al. 1986; Grossman et al. 1986b), while the effects of naloxone and CRF-41 are additive; this would suggest that the hypothalamic peptide(s) involved in both exogenous and endogenous responses is not CRF-41. Indeed, studies in the rat from our department indicate that the α_1- adrenoceptor regulation of ACTH occurs principally via vasopressin (S. Al-Damluji, unpublished observations), which may be directly subject to opioid inhibition. The nature of the endogenous opioid ligand is uncertain, but the relative resistance to naloxone and inference from extensive animal studies on neurohypophyseal vasopressin strongly implicate dynorphin-like peptides acting at κ-receptors (Van Wimersma Greidanus and Grossman 1990).

There is, however, evidence that CRF-41 is also involved in the opioid modulation of ACTH. While it is difficult to extrapolate from rat to human, particularly as the *acute* effect of opiates in the rat (as well as the sheep and the dog) is *stimulation* of the H-P-A axis, chronic treatment with morphine leads to pituitary-adrenal suppression (Briggs and Munson 1955). We have recently shown that the release of CRF-41 from the rat hypothalamus in vitro is also subject to opioid inhibition (Tsagarakis et al. 1989), with evidence implicating both μ-and κ-receptors (Fig. 3), but not δ- receptors, in this process (Tsagarakis et al. 1990). Interestingly enough, the μ-receptors appear to be rather insensitive to naloxone, as they do in the human. The acute stimulatory effects of opiates seen in subprimate species do not appear to directly involve CRF-41 (Nikolarakis et al. 1987; Cover and Buckingham 1989) and may relate to putative ACTH-inhibitory factors (?ANP/?MCH — see Grossman and Tsagarakis 1989).

Conclusions

In humans, the sympatho-adrenomedullary axis is subject to phasic opioid inhibition when activated, while the H-P-A axis is under tonic suppression. In both cases, the inhibition is relatively resistant to naloxone, and there are grounds for believing that the κ-subtype of opiate receptors is involved in these processes. For the H-P-A axis, this control probably occurs at several intrahypothalamic sites, involving vasopressin, CRF-41, and possibly other factors. For the sympathetic nervous system, the nucleus tractus solitarius in the brain-stem is a prime candidate for opioid interactions, but other more distal locations, such as the adrenal medulla (Jarry et al. 1989), cannot be excluded. Unravelling these counter-stress opioidergic systems may play an important part in understanding and treating the long-term deleterious consequences of stress.

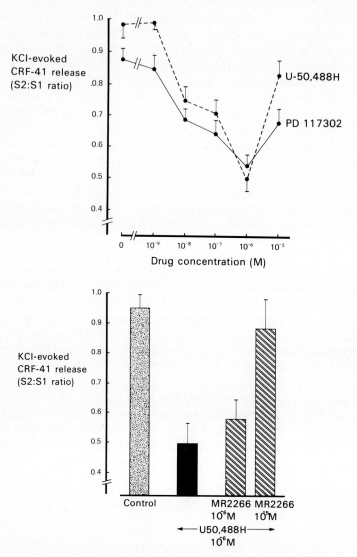

Fig. 3. *Upper panel:* The ratio of CRF-41 released from the rat hypothalamus in vitro following two successive incubations with 28 mmol/l KCl, in the absence (S1) or presence (S2) of a κ-receptor opiate agonist, *U-50,488H* or *PD 117302*. Each point represents the mean ± SEM. Note that the opiate agonists led to the inhibition of stimulated CRF-41 release, with maximal potencies at 1 μmol. *Lower panel:* As upper, but showing blockade of the inhibition produced by *U-50,488H* with the specific κ-receptor antagonist, *MR 2266*. (From Tsagarakis et al. 1990)

References

Al-Damluji S, Cunnah D, Grossman AB, Perry L, Ross G, Coy D, Rees LH, Besser GM (1987) Effect of adrenaline on basal and ovine corticotrophin releasing factor-stimulated ACTH secretion in man. J Endocrinol 112: 144-150

Allolio B, Winkelmann W, Hipp FX, Kaulen D, Miess R (1982) Effects of a met-enkephalin analog on adrenocorticotropin (ACTH), growth hormone and prolactin in patients with ACTH hypersecretion. J Clin Endocrinol Metab 55: 1-7

Allolio B, Deuss U, Kaulen D, Leonhardt U, Kallabis D, Hamel E, Winkelmann W (1986) FK 33-824, a met-enkephalin analog, blocks corticotropin-releasing hormone-induced adrenocorticotropin secretion in normal subjects but not in patients with Cushing's disease. J Clin Endocrinol Metab 63: 1427-1431

Bouloux PMG, Grossman A, Lytras N, Besser GM (1985) Evidence for the participation of endogenous opioids in the sympathoadrenal response to hypoglycaemia in man. Clin Endocrinol (Oxf) 22: 49-56

Bouloux PMG, Grossman A, Al-Damluji S, Bailey T, Besser GM (1986) Enhancement of the sympathoadrenal response to the cold pressor test by naloxone in man. Clin Sci 69: 365-368

Bouloux PMG, Grossman A (1989) Opioid involvement in the neuroendocrine response to stress in humans. In: Weiner H, Florin I, Murison R, Hellhammer D (eds) Frontiers of stress research. Huber, Toronto, pp 209-222

Bouloux PMG, Newbould E, Causon R, Perry L, Rees LH, Besser GM, Grossman A (1989) Differential effect of high-dose naloxone on the plasma adrenaline response to the cold-pressor test. Clin Sci 76: 625-630

Briggs FN, Munson PL (1955) Studies on the mechanism of stimulation of ACTH secretion with the aid of morphine as a blocking agent. Endocrinology 57: 205-219

Cover PO, Buckingham JC (1989) Effects of selective opioid- receptor blockade on the hypothalamo-pituitary-adrenocortical response to surgical trauma in the rat. J Endocrinol 121: 213-220

Delitala G, Grossman A, Besser M (1983) Differential effects of opiate peptides and alkaloids on anterior pituitary hormone secretion. Neuroendocrinology 37: 275-279

Drew JH, Drips RD, Comroe JH (1946) Clinical studies on morphine. The effect of morphine on the circulation in man and upon the circulatory and respiratory responses to tilting. Anesthesiology 7: 44-61

Gaillard RC, Grossman A, Smith R, Rees LH, Besser GM (1981) The effects of a met-enkephalin analogue on ACTH, β-LPH, β-endorphin and met-enkephalin in patients with adrenocortical disease. Clin Endocrinol (Oxf) 14: 471-478

Grossman A, Milles J, Baylis PH, Besser GM (1980) Inhibition of vasopressin release by an opiate peptide in man. Lancet ii: 1108- 1110

Grossman A, Smith R, Van Loon GR, Brown GM, Rees LH, Besser GM (1982a) Circulating catecholamines, melatonin and enkephalins in man following a met-enkephalin analogue. Neuroendocrinol Lett 4: 223-232

Grossman A, Gaillard RC, McCarthy P, Rees LH, Besser GM (1982b) Opiate modulation of the pituitary-adrenal axis: effects of stress and circadian rhythm. Clin Endocrinol (Oxf) 17: 279-286

Grossman A, Besser GM (1982) Opiates control ACTH through a noradrenergic mechanism. Clin Endocrinol (Oxf) 17: 287-290

Grossman A, Bouloux P, Price P, Drury P, Lam K, Turner T, Besser GM, Sutton J (1984) The role of opioid peptides in the hormonal responses to acute exercise. Clin Sci 67: 483-491

Grossman A, Moult PJA, Cunnah D, Besser GM (1986a) Different opioid mechanisms are involved in the modulation of gonadotrophin and ACTH release in man. Neuroendocrinology 42: 357-360

Grossman A, Delitala G, Coy DH, Besser GM (1986b) An analogue of met-enkephalin attenuates the cortisol response to ovine corticotrophin releasing factor. Clin Endocrinol (Oxf) 25: 421- 426

Grossman A, Tsagarakis S (1989) The hunt for the CIA: factors which demonstrate cor-ticotrophin-inhibitory activity. J Endocrinol 123: 169-172

Jarry H, Dietrich M, Barthel A, Giesler A, Wuttke W (1989) In vivo demonstration of a paracrine inhibitory action of met- enkephalin on adrenomedullary catecholamine release in the rat. Endocrinology 125: 624-629

Lam K, Grossman A, Bouloux P, Drury PL, Besser GM (1986) Effect of an opiate antagonist on the response of circulating catecholamines and the renin-aldosterone system to acute sympathetic stimulation by handgrip in man. Acta Endocrinol (Copenh) 111: 252-257

McCubbin JA, Surwit RS, Williams RB (1985) Endogenous opiate peptides, stress reactivity and risk for hypertension. Hypertension 7: 808-811

McDonald RK, Evans FT, Weise VK, Patrick RW (1959) Effect of morphine and nalorphine on plasma hydrocortisone levels in man. J Pharmacol Exp Ther 5: 241-247

Morris M, Salmon P, Steinberg H, Sykes EA, Bouloux P, McLoughlin L, Newbould E, Besser GM, Grossman A (1990) Endogenous opioids modulate the cardiovascular response to mental stress. Psychoneuroendocrinology (in press)

Nikolarakis K, Pfeiffer A, Stalla GK, Herz A (1987) The role of CRF in the release of ACTH by opiate agonists and antagonists in rats. Brain Res 421: 373-376

Rubin PC (1984) Opioid peptides in blood pressure regulation in man. Clin Sci 66: 625-630

Taylor T, Dluhy RG, Williams GH (1983) β-Endorphin suppresses adrenocorticotropin and cortisol levels in normal human subjects. J Clin Endocrinol Metab 57: 592-596

Tsagarakis S, Navara P, Rees LH, Besser GM, Grossman A (1989) Morphine directly modulates the release of stimulated corticotrophin releasing factor-41 from rat hypothalamus in vitro. Endocrinology 124: 2330-2335

Tsagarakis S, Rees LH, Besser GM, Grossman A (1990) Opiate receptor sub-type regulation of CRF-41 release from rat hypothalamus in vitro. Neuroendocrinology 51: 599-605

Van Wimersma Greidanus TB, Grossman A (1990) Opioid regulation of pituitary function. In: Ottoson D (ed) Progress in sensory physiology, vol 2. Springer, Berlin Heidelberg New York (in press)

Zelis R, Mansour EJ, Capoul RJ, Mason DT (1974) The cardiovascular effects of morphine. The peripheral capacitance and resistance vessels in the human subject. J Clin Invest 54: 1247-1258

Vasopressin: An Integrator of Proopiomelanocortin Activity in Brain and Pituitary

V.M. WIEGANT and C.G.J. SWEEP

Proopiomelanocortin

β-Endorphin (βE) and related peptides are synthesized as components of the multifactorial precursor molecule proopiomelanocortin (POMC), which also functions as the prohormone for corticotropin (ACTH), and melanotropin (α - MSH). Like ACTH and α-MSH, βE is liberated from this precursor molecule by proteolytic cleavage (Mains et al. 1977; Herbert et al. 1980). In the rat, POMC is synthesized in a variety of tissues including the corticotroph cells of the anterior lobe and the melanotroph cells of the intermediate lobe of the pituitary gland (Mains et al. 1977; Mains and Eipper 1979; Herbert et al. 1980). In the brain, POMC-containing neuronal cell bodies have been identified in different loci. The major cell group is located in the arcuate nucleus of the mediobasal hypothalamus (Watson et al. 1977; Bloom et al. 1978). Additional groups of neurons are found in the caudal part of the nucleus of the tractus solitarius (NTS) and in the nucleus commisuralis (Khachaturian et al. 1985; Palkovits et al. 1987). Numerous studies using immunocytochemical and bio-chemical techniques have dealt with the anatomy of these POMC-containing neuronal systems, and a wide array of brain structures appears to be innervated by POMC neurons (Watson et al. 1977; Finley et al. 1981). In particular, the POMC neurons in the arcuate nucleus form extensive projections to limbic and midbrain regions, whereas those found in the NTS area are thought to innervate primarily regions in the brainstem (Khachaturian et al. 1985; Palkovits et al. 1987). POMC-derived neuropeptides (including βE) can be secreted at the synaptic endings of these neurons, to act as neurotransmitters or neuromodu-lators and alter neuronal activity in a variety of brain circuits. As such, these peptides are involved in the regulation in the brain of cognitive, autonomous, and endocrine functions (O'Donohue and Dorsa 1982). In view of the different-ing and often antagonistic activities in this respect of peptides related to ACTH/α-MSH and βE, POMC may be viewed as a multifactorial controller of homeostatic functions (de Wied 1987).

POMC-Derived Peptides in the Cerebrospinal Fluid

The presence of peptides derived from POMC has been demonstrated in brain tissue as well as in the cerebrospinal fluid (CSF) of the rat (Kiser et al. 1983; Jackson et al. 1985; C.G.J. Sweep and V.M. Wiegant, unpublished results). Although no direct axonal projections of POMC neurons to the ventricles have been described sofar, the results of many studies indicate that peptide levels in plasma and CSF are under separate regulation, and that the neuropeptides found in the CSF probably originate from cells in the brain rather than from the pituitary. It has been shown for instance, that hypophysectomy does not affect the concentration of POMC-derived peptides in the CSF (de Rotte et al. 1986), and that under a variety of experimental conditions no correlation exists between their concentration in the CSF and in plasma (de Rotte et al. 1982; Barna et al. 1988). Moreover, electrical stimulation of brain regions containing POMC neurons or fibers results in increased levels of βE in the CSF (Akil et al. 1978). The ventricular CSF forms a continuum with the extracellular fluid in the brain, and neuropeptides, once released at synapses in the brain, may reach the CSF by diffusion or by drainage of extracellular fluid into the ventricular compartment. The concentration of neuropeptides in the CSF is thus a function of secretory activity of brain neurons. In addition, clearance mechanisms are operative in the CSF, and constitute an additional factor that determines peptide concentrations in CSF. As CSF contains no significant proteolytic activity to convert endorphins (Burbach et al. 1979), the clearance of these neuropeptides from the CSF likely depends on their transport from the ventricular system to other compartments, e.g., to blood or brain tissue.

Release of βE-Derived Peptides from Pituitary and Brain

The regulation of the secretory activity of POMC cells in the pituitary has been well investigated. The anterior lobe of the pituitary gland is highly vascularized and not innervated. As a consequence, the release of POMC-derived peptides from this lobe is controlled by humoral factors, mainly from the hypothalamus. This regulation is a multifactorial process and apart from corticotropin-releasing hormone (CRH), it involves other hypothalamic peptides, such as vasopressin. Vasopressin and CRH are both synthesized by neurons located in the paraventricularis nucleus of the hypothalamus and secreted from nerve terminals in the external zone of the median eminence into the portal circulation, via which they can reach the anterior lobe of the pituitary gland (for review see Jones and Gillham 1988). In contrast to the corticotrophs, the activity of pituitary melanotrophs is mainly regulated by direct neural input from the hypothalamus. Dopaminergic nerve fibers, originating in the nucleus arcuatus and projecting directly to the melanotrophs, are the main — inhibitory — controllers of the activity of these POMC cells, whereas catecholamines of adrenomedullary origin are probably responsible for β-adrenoceptor mediated stimulation of peptide secretion by the intermediate lobe (Tilders et al. 1975; Cote et al. 1980).

In contrast to our knowledge of the pituitary gland, little information is available on the regulation of the secretory activity of POMC neuronal cells in the brain. In a series of studies, we therefore addressed the question whether or not the same principles are involved in the regulation of the secretory activity of pituitary and brain POMC cells. Since the CSF is a relatively readily accessible compartment of the brain, and the concentration of peptides in the CSF is representative for the peptide climate in the brain, we used in these studies the βE level in CSF, determined by radioimmunoassay, as an index for POMC cell activity in the brain. We studied the effects of intracerebroventricular (i.c.v.) injection of CRH, arginine[8]-vasopressin (AVP), or the β-adrenoceptor agonist isoproterenol, well known pituitary secretagogues, on the concentration of βE-immunoreactivity in the CSF. It was found that AVP dose-dependently induces changes in the concentration of βE-immunoreactivity in the CSF, whereas isoproterenol and CRH were ineffective in this respect (Barna et al. 1990; Sweep 1989; Sweep et al. 1990).

Dual Effects of Vasopressin on the Concentration of βE-Immunoreactivity in the CSF

Vasopressin Enhances the Clearance of βE from the CSF

Intracerebroventricular administration of AVP in doses of 0.1 and 1 pg per rat induces a decrease in the concentration of βE-immunoreactivity in CSF withdrawn 5 min after treatment, as compared to vehicle-treated controls (Fig.1), whereas 10 pg AVP is not active in this respect. This effect is of short duration and no significant changes in CSF endorphin levels are found 10 and 20 min after AVP treatment.

As argued, the concentration of βE-immunoreactivity in the CSF is determined by the secretory activity of βE-producing neuronal cells in the brain and by the clearance of βE from the ventricular compartments. The decrease in CSF βE-immunoreactivity levels following intracerebroventricular treatment of rats with 0.1 and 1 pg AVP could thus be brought about by a decreased release of βE from brain stores, or an enhanced clearance of βE from the CSF, or both. In view of the apparent half-life of βE in rat CSF (which is approximately 29 min; Sweep et al. 1990), it is not likely that a decreased release of βE and related peptides underlies this effect of AVP, for even a complete blockade of their release could not account for the 30% decrease in βE-immunoreactivity levels 5 min after AVP administration. Moreover, it appeared that treatment of rats with AVP (i.c.v., 1 pg) also accelerates the disappearance of intracerebroventricularly injected synthetic βE from the CSF (Fig. 2). The CSF does not

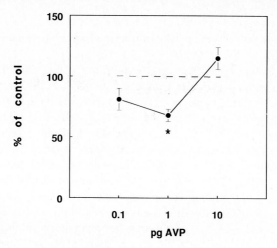

Fig. 1. Effect of intracerebroventricular (i.c.v.) injection of AVP on the concentration of βE-immunoreactivity in CSF. Male rats were equipped with two permanent cannulas, one ending in the lateral brain ventricle, used for i.c.v. injection (3 μl) of substances, and another ending in the cisterna magna, allowing repeated withdrawal of CSF (40-100 μl) from the conscious animal. CSF was collected 5 min after i.c.v. injection of 0.1 -10 pg AVP. The concentration of βE- immunoreactivity in the CSF was determined by radioimmunoassay using an antiserum recognizing the midportion of the βE (1-31) molecule (see Barna et al. 1988). Data are expressed as percentage of the mean βE-immunoreactivity values in vehicle-injected control rats, and presented as mean ± SEM ($n = 8–10$). A treatment × dose effect was observed [$F(3,4) = 5.2$; $p < 0.003$; one-way analysis of variance (ANOVA) followed by Student-Newman Keuls (SNK) test]. *, p (Student's t test)

contain enzymes capable of degrading βE. Therefore, the AVP-induced decrease in the concentration of βE-immunoreactivity in CSF is likely caused by an increase in the clearance rate of endorphins from the ventricular system.

In view of the extremely low active dose of AVP and the route of administration, it is likely that AVP induces its effect by an action on structures within the brain. Structure activity studies showing that fragments of AVP and the structurally related peptides oxytocin and lysine[8]-vasopressin are inactive in lowering the concentration of βE in CSF when intracerebroventricularly injected in a dose of 1 pg (Sweep et al. 1990), suggest that specific vasopressin receptors are involved. The vasopressin receptors in the central nervous system appear to be predominantly of the V_1 subtype (Tribollet et al. 1988). Indeed, intracerebroventricular pretreatment of rats with the vasopressin V_1 receptor antagonist d(CH2)5Tyr(Me)AVP completely blocks the effect of AVP on CSF βE-immunoreactivity levels (Sweep et al. 1990; Sweep 1989). Binding sites for vasopressin have been found on cerebral microvessels (van Zwieten et al. 1988) and on the choroid plexus (Van Leeuwen et al., 1987), suggesting that vasopressin may be involved in the regulation of fluid transport across membranes in the brain. Therefore, we cannot rule out the possibility that changes in the brain's

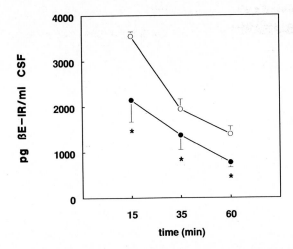

Fig. 2. Effect of AVP on the clearance from the CSF of i.c.v. administered synthetic βE. Rats were i.c.v. injected with 5 ng βE (1-31) and 10, 30, and 55 min later with vehicle (*open circles*) or 1 pg AVP (*closed circles*). CSF was collected 5 min later. Data are expressed as pg βE- immunoreactivity per ml CSF and represent the mean ± SEM of 6-11 observations. *, Significantly different from the vehicle- treated controls (ANOVA followed by SNK)

water balance underly or contribute to the effect of AVP on the concentration of βE-immunoreactivity in the CSF.

Vasopressin Stimulates the Release of βE from Brain Tissue

Intracerebroventricular injection of rats with AVP in doses of 10-1000 pg induces a dose-dependent increase in the concentration of βE-immunoreactivity in the CSF (see Fig. 3). This effect appears to be time-dependent and reaches its maximum 20-35 min after treatment (Barna et al. 1990). Following the same line of reasoning as for the inhibitory effect of AVP on CSF endorphin levels, this AVP-induced increase might be the result of a stimulatory action of the peptide on the secretory activity of POMC neurons in the brain, or an inhibitory action on the clearance of βE and related peptides from the CSF, or both. In view of the half-life of βE in the CSF (Sweep et al. 1990), even a complete blockade of the clearance would not account for the observed increase in βE-immunoreactivity in the CSF within 10 min. Therefore, the observed effect of AVP is interpreted as evidence for a stimulatory action of the peptide on the release of βE from cells in the brain.

Pretreatment (i.c.v.) of rats with the V_1 vasopressin receptor antagonist (1ng) completely inhibited the effect of the peptide (100 pg). The involvement of a V_1-type vasopressin receptor is also indicated by the structure-activity relationships found (Sweep 1989; Sweep et al., in preparation). Interestingly, the

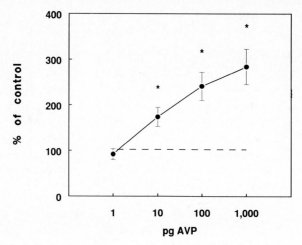

Fig. 3. Effect of i.c.v. injection of AVP on the concentration of βE-immunoreactivity in CSF. The CSF was collected 20 min after treatment. Data are expressed as percentage of the mean βE-immunoreactivity values in vehicle- treated control rats, and are shown as mean ± SEM ($n = 6$–15). A treatment [$F(1,4)=36.4$; p], dose [$F(3,4)=27.3$; p], and treatment × dose [$F (3,4) = 5.2$; p] effect of AVP was found (ANOVA). *, p versus vehicle-treated controls (Student's t test)

stimulatory effect of AVP on CSF βE levels is also observed upon subcutaneous administration of the peptide, but much higher doses (3-5 μg) are needed than with the intracerebroventricular route. Intracerebroventricular pretreatment with low doses of the V_1 receptor antagonist (10 ng) completely blocks this peripheral effect, further evidencing the central site of action of AVP in this respect (Sweep 1989; Sweep et al., in preparation).

The question then arises where in the brain the sites responsible for the stimulatory effect of AVP on CSF βE-immunoreactivity levels are located. Circumstantial evidence points toward the mediobasal hypothalamus as a possible site of action, as (a) this area contains cell bodies of POMC neurons, and binding sites for the vasopressor antagonist d (CH$_2$) $_5$ Tyr (Me) AVP (Finley et al. 1977; van Leeuwen et al. 1987) and (b) intracerebroventricular administration of AVP to rats alters the concentration of βE-immunoreactivity in the hypothalamus (I. Barna and V.M. Wiegant, unpublished results). A vasopressinergic control of hypothalamic POMC cells is further supported by observations that electrical lesions of the paraventricularis and supraoptic nuclei results in marked changes in the βE content of the hypothalamus (Millan et al. 1983, 1984).

To obtain direct evidence for an action of vasopressin on the secretory activity of βE-containing neuronal cells in the brain, the effect of AVP on the release of βE and related peptides from rat hypothalamic tissue in vitro was studied (Sweep and Wiegant 1989). As shown in Fig. 4, AVP stimulates in a

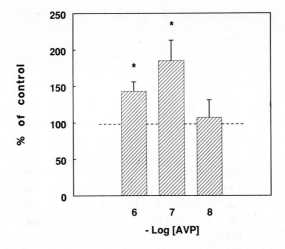

Fig. 4. Effect of AVP on the release of βE-immunoreactivity from rat hypothalamic tissue in vitro. For procedure see Sweep and Wiegant (1989). The data represent the concentration of βE-immunoreactivity in incubation media after exposure for 30 min of hypothalamic fragments to different concentrations of AVP, and are expressed as percentage of the amount of βE-immunoreactivity released during parallel incubations of tissue fragments with control medium. Means ± SEM of 4-5 observations are presented. * Significant difference vs. control (p; Student's t test)

concentration-dependent manner the release of βE-immunoreactivity from mediobasal hypothalamic tissue fragments, indeed suggesting that vasopressin may regulate the activity of central POMC neurons at the level of the hypothalamus.

Vasopressin in Rat Brain and the Diurnal Rhythm of βE-Immunoreactivity in CSF

Vasopressin is synthesized in several groups of neuronal cells in the brain, and in addition to being secreted from the neurohypophysis functions as a neuropeptide in the brain. The data reviewed above suggest that endogenous vasopressin fullfills a role as neuropeptide regulator of the activity of hypothalamic POMC cells. An interesting question now pertains to the origin of this vasopressin.

Vasopressin synthesizing neurons can be distinguished into magnocellular and parvocellular neurons. Magnocellular vasopressin neurons are found in the supraoptic nucleus, PVN and in the accessory nuclei. Nearly all of these cells project to the posterior lobe of the pituitary gland, from which vasopressin is secreted into the circulation. Parvocellular vasopressin neurons are located in the paraventricularis nucleus, the suprachiasmatic nucleus, and in some extrahypothalamic brain regions such as the bed nucleus of the stria terminalis.

Although the anatomy of these vasopressin systems is not yet completely elucidated, parvocellular neurons are known to project in various regions of the brain (Buys 1987). Thus, the suprachiasmatic nucleus is among the possible sites where vasopressin impinging on POMC neurons may originate. This nucleus is the locus of a circadian pacemaker that generates hormonal rhythms, including that of vasopressin in the CSF (Reppert et al. 1987). In the rat, vasopressin levels in CSF are highest during the light period and low at the end of the light and during the dark period. In order to probe whether vasopressin derived from the suprachiasmatic nucleus is involved in the regulation of βE release in the brain, we studied the βE-immunoreactivity levels in the CSF of rats at various times during the day–night cycle. The results are presented in Fig. 5 and show that the concentration of βE-immunoreactivity in the CSF exhibits a complex 24 h rhythmicity. From the onset of the dark period, βE levels gradually increase, reaching peak values at 2.00 am of approximately 1000 pg/ml. Thereafter, βE-immunoreactivity levels declined to approximately 500 pg/ml at 4.00 a.m. and 6.00 am, when the lights were switched on. Two hours later, a sharp peak was found, while during the remainder of the light period the concentration of βE-immunoreactivity remained at a stable basal level of around 500 pg/ml. This diurnal rhythm of βE clearly differs from that reported for vasopressin in the CSF. This suggests, that vasopressin originating from the suprachiasmatic nucleus is not a major factor in the regulation of the βE concentration in CSF.

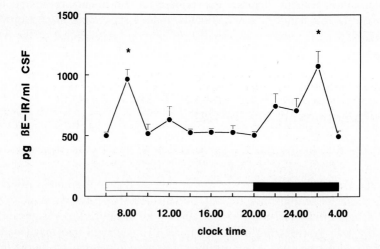

Fig. 5. CSF levels of βE-immunoreactivity (pg/ml) at various time points during the day–night cycle. Rats were kept under a normal regulat 14 h light – 10 h dark regimen of illumination (lights on at 06.00 h). Data are presented as pg βE-immunoreactivity per ml CSF and represent the mean ± SEM of 5–10 observations [$F(11,88) = 6.54$; p]

Concluding Remarks

AVP appears to be an extremely potent modulator of the βE concentration in the CSF. By interaction with specific receptors located in the central nervous system, the peptide induces two types of effects with different dose–response and time–effect relationships: (1) enhancement of the clearance of βE from the CSF, and (2) stimulation of the release of βE from stores in the hypothalamus. This suggests that endogenous vasopressin is involved in the regulation of the POMC-peptide milieu in the brain.

Peptides derived from POMC are secreted by the pituitary into the circulation, to convey their message as peptide hormones to distant peripheral target tissues. They are also released by brain neurons to act as neurotransmitters or neuromodulators and influence neuronal activity at different sites in the central nervous system. In either case, they are liberated upon stressful challenge and are believed to serve the adaptation of the organism to potentially harmful changes in the internal and external milieu. Based on the data reviewed, we suggest that, in addition to its well-known function as a releasing hormone for pituitary POMC-derived peptide hormones, vasopressin is a releaser of POMC-derived neuropeptides in the brain. Thus, vasopressin, liberated under stressful conditions from neurons in the hypothalamus, may integrate central and peripheral adaptive responses to stress that are mediated by peptides derived from POMC.

References

Akil H, Richardson DE, Barchas JD, Li CH (1978) Appearance of β-endorphin-like immunoreactivity in human ventricular cerebrospinal fluid upon analgesic electrical stimulation. Proc Natl Acad Sci USA 75: 5170-5172

Barna I, Sweep CGJ, Veldhuis HD, Wiegant VM (1988) Differential effects of cisterna magna cannulation on β-endorphin levels in rat plasma and cerebrospinal fluid. Acta Endocrinol (Copenh) 117: 517-524

Barna I, Sweep CGJ, Veldhuis HD, Wiegant VM, de Wied D (1990) Effects of pituitary β-endorphin secretagogues on the concentration of β-endorphin in rat cerebrospinal fluid: evidence for a role of vasopressin in the regulation of brain β-endorphin. Neuroendocrinology 51: 104-110

Bloom F, Battenberg E, Rossier J, Ling N, Guillemin R (1978) Neurons containing beta-endorphin in rat brain exist separately from those containing enkephalin: immunocytochemical studies. Proc Natl Acad Sci USA 75: 1591-1595

Burbach JPH, Loeber JG, Verhoef J, de Kloet ER, van Ree JM, de Wied D (1979) Schizophrenia and degradation of endorphins in cerebrospinal fluid. Lancet 1: 480-481

Buys RM (1987) Vasopressin localisation and putative functions in the brain. In: Gash DM, Boer GJ (eds) Vasopressin; principles and properties. Plenum, New York, pp 91-115

Cote T, Munemura M, Eskay RL, Kebabian JW (1980) Biochemical identification of the β-adrenoceptor and evidence for the involvement of an adenosine 3'5'-monophosphate system in the β-adrenergically induced release of α-melanocyte-stimulating hormone in the intermediate lobe of the rat pituitary gland. Endocrinology 107: 108-116

De Rotte AA, van Wimersma Greidanus TB (1982) Differential secretion of α-melanocyte stimulating hormone into cerebrospinal fluid and blood in the rat. Front Horm Res Vol 9 131-141

De Rotte AA, Verhoef J, Andringa-Bakker EAD, van Wimersma Greidanus TB (1986) Characterization of the α-MSH-like immunoreactivity in blood and cerebrospinal fluid of the rat. Acta Endocrinol (Copen) 111: 440-444

De Wied D (1987) The neuropeptide concept. Prog Brain Res 72: 93-108

Finley JCW, Lindström P, Petrusz P (1981) Immunocytochemical localization of β-endorphin-containing neurons in the rat brain. Neuroendocrinology 33: 28-42

Herbert E, Roberts J, Phillips M, Allen R, Hinman M, Budarf M, Policastro P, Rosa P (1980) Biosynthesis, processing, and release of corticotropin, β-endorphin, and melanocyte stimulating hormone in pituitary cell culture systems. In: Martini L, Canoung WF (eds) Frontiers in neuroendocrinology. Raven, New York, pp 67-101

Jackson S, Kiser S, Corder R, Lowry PJ (1985) Pro-opiocortin peptides in rat cerebrospinal fluid. Regul Pept 11: 159-171

Jones MT, Gillham B (1988) Factors involved in the regulation of adrenocorticotropic hormone/β-lipotropic hormone. Physiol Rev 68: 743-818

Khachaturian H, Lewis ME, Tsou K, Watson SJ (1985) β- Endorphin, α-MSH, ACTH, and related peptides. In: Björklund A, Hökfelt T (eds) Handbook of chemical neuroanatomy, vol 4. Elsevier, Amsterdam, pp 216-272

Kiser RS, Jackson S, Smith R, Rees LH, Lowry PJ, Besser GM (1983) Endorphin-related peptides in rat cerebrospinal fluid. Brain Res 288: 187-192

Mains RE, Eipper BA, Ling N (1977) Common precursor to corticotropins and endorphins. Proc Natl Acad Sci USA 74: 3014-3018

Mains RE, Eipper BA (1979) Synthesis and secretion of corticotropins, melanotropins, and endorphins by rat intermediate pituitary cells. J Biol Chem 254: 7885-7894

Millan MJ, Millan MH, Herz A (1983) Contribution of the supra-optic nucleus to brain and pituitary pools of immunoreactive vasopressin and particular opioid peptides and the interrelationships between these in the rat. Neuroendocrinology 36: 310-319

Millan MH, Millan MJ, Herz A (1984) The hypothalamic paraventricular nucleus: relationship to brain and pituitary pools of vasopressin and oxytocin as compared to dynorphin β-endorphin and related opioid peptides in the rat. Neuroendocrinology 38: 108-116

O'Donohue TL, Dorsa DM (1982) The opiomelanotropinergic neuronal and endocrine systems. Peptides 3: 353

Palkovits M, Me/zey E, Eskay RL (1987) Pro-opiomelanocortin derived peptides (ACTH/β-endorphin/α-MSH) in brainstem baroreceptor areas of the rat. Brain Res 436: 323-328

Reppert SM, Schwartz WJ, Uhl GR (1987) Arginine vasopressin: a novel rhythm in cerebrospinal fluid. Top Neurol Sci 109: 76-80

Sweep CGJ (1989) Studies on the regulation of β-endorphin producing cells in rat brain and pituitary. Thesis, University of Utrecht

Sweep CGJ, Wiegant VM (1989) Release of β-endorphin-immunoreactivity from rat pituitary and hypothalamus in vitro: effects of isoproterenol, dopamine, corticotropin-releasing factor and arginine[8]-vasopressin. Biochem Biophys Res Commun 161: 221-228

Sweep CGJ, Boomkamp MD, Barna I, Logtenberg AW, Wiegant VM (1989) Vasopressin enhances the clearance of β-endorphin-immunoreactivity from rat cerebrospinal fluid. Acta Endocrinol (Copenh) 122: 191-200

Tilders FJH, Mulder AH, Smelik PG (1975) On the presence of a MSH-release inhibiting system in the rat neurointermediate lobe. Neuroendocrinology 18: 125-130

Tribollet E, Barberis C, Jard S, Dubois-Dauphin M, Dreifuss JJ (1988) Localization and pharmacological characterization of high affinity binding sites for vasopressin and oxytocin in the rat brain by light microscopic autoradiography. Brain Res 442: 105-108

Van Leeuwen FW, van Der Beek EM, van Heerikhuize JJ, Wolters P, van der Meulen G, Wan YP (1987) Quantitative light microscopic autoradiographic localization of binding sites labelled with [^{3}H] vasopressin antagonist d (CH$_2$) 5 Tyr (Me) VP in the rat brain, pituitary and kidney. Neurosci Lett 80: 121-126

Van Zwieten EJ, Ravid R, Swaab DF, van der Woude T (1988) Immunocytochemically stained vasopressin binding sites on blood vessels in the rat brain. Brain Res 474: 369-373

Watson SJ, Barchas JD, Li CH (1977) β-Lipotropin: localization of cells and axons in rat brain by immunocytochemistry. Proc Natl Acad Sci USA 74: 5155-5158

β-Endorphin Immunoreactive Material in the Plasma: What Does It Mean?

H. TESCHEMACHER, G. KOCH, D. KRAMER, and K. WIEDEMANN

The Problem

During the last decade, much information has been collected on the biosynthesis, structure, distribution, and effects of opioid peptides; however, our knowledge about the physiological significance of these peptides has still remained marginal (Illes and Farsang 1988).

To understand the functional relevance of β-endorphin in plasma, or to understand the mechanisms of physiological or pathological states or drug effects, many studies have been performed searching for an interrelationship between β-endorphin levels in plasma and such states or effects; in Table 1 a number of arbitrarily chosen studies are given.

Basically, the aim was to obtain data as to whether the β-endorphin concentration in the plasma might play any role in connection with the "parameter"

Table 1. Studies in which the possible interrelationship between plasma levels of β-endorphin immunoreactive material and, a variety of "parameters", i.e. physiological or pathological states etc. are investigated

Parameter	Reference
Hypovolemic shock	Daly et al. (1987)
Primary aldosteronism	Griffing et al. (1985)
Menopausal hot flushes	Tepper et al. (1987)
Heroin addiction	Facchinetti et al. (1985)
Physical stress	Elias et al. (1989)
Polycystic ovarian disease	Nappi et al. (1989)
Depressive states	Weizman et al. (1987)
Rheumatic disorders	Denko et al. (1986)
Water immersion	Coruzzi et al. (1988)
"Runner's high"	Wildmann et al. (1986)
Pregnancy	Räisänen (1988)
Drug effect (cortisol)	Bagdy et al. (1989)
Male infertility	Miralles-Garcia et al. (1986)

studied. However, the only way to obtain this information appeared to be to determine the concentration of β-endorphin immunoreactive material in plasma in parallel and to look for the parameter studied. Transformation of the question: "Does β-endorphin in the plasma play a role in connection with the parameter..." into "Is β-endorphin released into the systemic circulation to carry a message from a trigger to an effector system functionally related to the 'parameter'..." (since how else could one interpret an increase of the β-endorphin level in plasma?) immediately elucidates the situation: one just has to ask oneself whether the experimental design usually chosen for determination of β-endorphin immunoreactive material in the plasma is in fact able to provide an answer to the expanded question, which takes the given biological situation in the organism into account. To cut it short: Does the method fit the concept? To ascertain this, one has to ask:

1. Does β-endorphin immunoreactive material correspond to β-endorphin?
2. Does the plasma concentration of β-endorphin immunoreactive material reflect the concentration of β-endorphin released into the cardiovascular compartment?
3. Does the plasma concentration of β-endorphin immunoreactive material reflect the message from trigger to effector system?
4. Does determination of the plasma concentration of β-endorphin immunoreactive material give information about any functional interrelationship between the "parameter" studied (e.g., stress) and any trigger or effector system?
— i.e., where does β-endorphin immunoreactive material come from, and where does it go to?

In the present article a critical evaluation of findings will be given which might help to answer these four questions.

Immunoreactive Material: A Material with a Defined Identity ?

As can be seen from the literature (Frederickson and Geary 1982), there is great variation in the levels of β-endorphin immunoreactive material determined in the plasma under normal conditions; in addition, more materials than just β-endorphin and β-LPH have been found in several studies.

Assuming that methodological differences were the cause of these discrepancies, we developed a method (Wiedemann and Teschemacher 1986) which ought to give clear cut and reproducible results.

Acidified EDTA plasma was extracted using an octadecasilyl cartridge adsorption/desorption technique and the extracts were subjected to a multiple radioimmunoassay system. In this radioimmunoassay system samples were analyzed using three antisera directed against different segments of the β-endorphin molecule, in order to ascertain whether the whole β-endorphin molecule and not only a certain segment is present in the sample (usually one antiserum is used only). Where there was a positive result the extracts were subjected to high-pressure liquid chromatography and the eluates again analyzed by multiple radioimmunoassay.

The method was applied to plasma samples from healthy volunteers (controls), volunteers under physical/emotional stress (free climbers), volunteers undergoing stimulation of the immune system (after vaccination, etc.), and patients suffering from immunological or neoplastic diseases (Kramer et al. 1988).

Strikingly, neither in healthy volunteers nor in patients were we able to detect authentic β-endorphin, except in a very few cases. In most subjects, immunoreactive material was recognized by one of the antisera but not by the other two, indicating that, instead of β-endorphin, just one of the β-endorphin segments or related materials were present in the sample. Thus, in our experience, although β-endorphin immunoreactive material can be found in most human plasma samples, this immunoreactivity does not appear to be β-endorphin in our studies — possibly not even a proopiomelanocortin (POMC) derivative.

Plasma: Representative of the Cardiovascular Compartment?

In most studies concentrations of immunoreactive β-endorphin were determined in plasma, since it is easier to handle than other components of the cardiovascular compartment. However, studies by Fisher et al. (1984) and Evans et al. (1985) clearly show that the erythrocyte compartment contains high amounts (to about the same magnitude as the plasma compartment) of β-endorphin immunoreactive material. This level varies from species to species and is different in normal and pathological states. This makes the plasma compartment an unreliable representative of the cardiovascular compartment which, in toto, is the carrier of the message released from any trigger system.

β-Endorphin Immunoreactive Material in Plasma: A Material with Clear-Cut Messenger Information?

β-Endorphin is a POMC cleavage product: However as shown in Table 2 — depending on the tissue in which the POMC gene is expressed — the number of β-endorphin derivatives varies between five and eight peptides (Smyth 1983; Cheng et al. 1985; Lolait et al. 1986; Höllt 1986). An antiserum directed against the N-terminal portion of the β-endorphin molecule usually would not be able to differentiate between the eight β-endorphin derivatives. Since the trigger system obviously has the possibility to release a very detailed message into the plasma, using from one to eight different compounds in quantities from zero to "physiologically preset" amounts, the determination of a nondifferentiated average concentration just counteracts "decoding" of the message; on the contrary, "misreading" is even a more likely consequence of this experimental design.

Table 2. Posttranslational POMC processing: β-endorphin and its derivatives; * presence in vivo to be confirmed

Pituitary(rat)	β-Endorphin	(1–31)	/	N–acetyl–β-endorphin	(1–31)
	β-Endorphin	(1–27)	/	N–acetyl–β-endorphin	(1–27)
	β-Endorphin	(1–26)	/	N–acetyl–β-endorphin	(1–26)
	*β-Endorphin	(1–17)	/	N–acetyl–β-endorphin	(1–17)
	*β-Endorphin	(1–16)			
Testis (rat)	β-Endorphin	(1–31)	/	N–acetyl–β-endorphin	(1–31)
				N–acetyl–β-endorphin	(1–27)
				N–acetyl–β-endorphin	(1–17)
				N–acetyl–β-endorphin	(1–16)
Spleen (mouse)	β-Endorphin	(1–31)	/	N–acetyl–β-endorphin	(1–31)
				N–acetyl–β-endorphin	(1–27)
				N–acetyl–β-endorphin	(1–17)
				N–acetyl–β-endorphin	(1–16)

β-Endorphin Immunoreactive Material in Plasma: A Reliable Correlate of the Functional State of a Trigger–Effector System?

There are a considerable number of cells or tissues in the organism where the POMC gene is expressed and from which, therefore, β-endorphin or its derivatives could be released, e.g. T- or B-cells, mass cells, macrophages, pituitary, testis, epididymis, seminal vesicles, ovary or placenta (Kavelaars et al. 1989; Evans et al. 1983; Chen et al. 1984, 1986; Piccoli et al. 1988; Zurawski et al. 1986; Lolait et al. 1984; Martin et al. 1987). Conclusive evidence for extrapituitary sources for β-endorphin or its derivatives in vivo has been published by several groups (Genazzani et al. 1988; Facchinetti et al. 1987; Kerdelhué et al. 1982).

There are also a considerable number of potential sites of action for β-endorphin and its derivatives when present in blood: in particular, sites provided by the immune system (Sibinga and Goldstein 1988), but also other tissues where the POMC gene is expressed (see above) for the respective short loops.

In view of this situation, it appears very difficult to obtain, from a measurement of the average β-endorphin/β-endorphin derivative concentration in the plasma, information about the source of the components of this mixture or the target they are destined for. The situation would not be much better even if the compounds were known.

Although it can give hints—in that, to our present knowledge, already very low concentrations are able to elicit effects on targets within the immune system—the β-endorphin immunoreactive material cannot be called a reliable indicator of changes in the particular functional state of a particular trigger–effector system.

Conclusion

The determination of β-endorphin immunoreactive material in the plasma has been a valuable tool in establishing a basis of information on interrelationships between on the one hand, a series of drug effects and physiological and pathological states in the organism and, on the other, part of the endogenous opioid peptidergic systems, i.e. β-endorphin in the plasma. At this stage, however, arguments relating to the complexity of the trigger–effector systems in the organism, and, in addition the stagnation of progress in the knowledge on this field, speak in favour of switching trails to more subtle experimental designs.

References

Bagdy G, Calogero AE, Chrousos GP, Szemeredi K (1989) Delayed effects of chronic cortisol treatment on brain and plasma concentrations of corticotropin (ACTH) and β-endorphin. Brain Res 489:216-222

Chen C-L, Mather JP, Morris PL, Bardin CW (1984) Expression of pro-opiomelanocortin-like gene in the testis and epididymis. Proc Natl Acad Sci USA 81:5672-5675

Chen C-L, Chang C-C, Krieger DR, Bardin CW (1986) Expression and regulation of proopiomelanocortin-like gene in the ovary and placenta: comparison with the testis. Endocrinology 118:2382-2389

Cheng MC, Clements JA, Smith AI, Lolait SJ, Funder JW (1985) N-acetyl-endorphin in rat spermatogonia and primary spermatocytes. J Clin Invest 75:832-835

Coruzzi P, Ravanetti C, Musiari L, Biggi A, Vescovi PP, Novarini A (1988) Circulating opioid peptides during water immersion in normal man. Clin Sci 74:133-136

Daly T, Beamer KC, Vargish T, Wilson A (1987) Correlation of plasma β-endorphin levels with mean arterial pressure and cardiac output in hypovolemic shock. Crit Care Med 15:723-725

Denko CW, Aponte J, Gabriel P, Petricevic M (1986) β- endorphin, immunological and biochemical changes in the synovial fluid in rheumatic disorders. Clin Rheumatol 5:25-32

Elias AN, Fairshter R, Pandian MR, Domurat E, Kayaleh R (1989) Lipotropin release and gonadotropin secretion after acute exercise in physically conditioned males. Eur J Appl Physiol 58:522-527

Evans MI, Fisher AM, Robichaux AG, Staton RC, Rodbard D, Larsen JW, Mukherjee AB (1985) Plasma and red blood cell β-endorphin immunoreactivity in normal and complicated pregnancies: gestational age variation. Am J Obstet Gynecol 151:433-437

Evans CJ, Erdelyi E, Weber E, Barchas JD (1983) Identification of pro-opiomelanocortin-derived peptides in the human adrenal medulla. Science 221:957-960

Facchinetti F, Livieri C, Petraglia F, Cortona L, Severi F, Genazzani AR (1987) Dexamethasone fails to suppress hyperendorphinaemia of obese children. Acta Endocrinol (Copenh) 116:90-94

Facchinetti F, Volpe A, Nappi G, Petraglia F, Genazzani AR (1985) Impairment of adrenergic-induced proopiomelanocortin-related peptide release in heroin addicts. Acta Endocrinol 108:1-5

Fisher A, Comly M, Do R, Tamarkin L, Ghazanfari AF, Mukherjee AB (1984) Two pools of β-endorphin-like immunoreactivity in blood: plasma and erythrocytes. Life Sci 34:1839-1846

Frederickson RCA, Geary LE (1982) Endogenous opioid peptides: review of physiological, pharmacological and clinical aspects. Prog Neurobiol 19:19-69

Genazzani AR, Petraglia F, Facchinetti F, Golinelli S, Oltramari P, Santoro V, Volpe A (1988) Evidences for a dopamine-regulated peripheral source of circulating β-endorphin. J Clin Endocrinol Metab 66:279-282

Griffing GT, McIntosh T, Berelowitz B, Hudson M, Salzman R, Manson JAE, Melby JC (1985) Plasma β-endorphin levels in primary aldosteronism. J Clin Endocrinol Metab 60:315-318

Höllt V (1986) Opioid peptide processing and receptor selectivity. Annu Rev Pharmacol Toxicol 26:59-77

Illes P, Farsang C (eds) (1988) Regulatory roles of opioid peptides. VCH, Basel

Kavelaars A, Ballieux RE, Heijnen CJ (1989) The role of IL-1 in the corticotropin-releasing factor and arginine-vasopressin-induced secretion of immunoreactive β-endorphin by human peripheral blood mononuclear cells. J Immunol 142:2338-2342

Kerdelhué B, Bethea CL, Ling N, Chrétien M, Weiner RI (1982) β-endorphin concentrations in serum, hypothalamus and central gray of hypophysectomized and mediobasal hypothalamus lesioned rats. Brain Res 231:85-91

Kramer D, Geiger L, Paul E, Breidenbach T, Wiedemann K, Teschemacher H (1988) "β-Endorphin immunoreactivity" in human plasma may consist of various compounds not identical with β- endorphin or β-LPH (Abstr. P 102). International Narcotics Research Conference, Albi, France, July 3-8, 1988

Lolait SJ, Clements JA, Markwick AJ, Cheng C, McNally M, Smith AI, Funder JW (1986) Pro-opiomelano-cortin messenger ribonucleic acid and posttranslational processing of β-endorphin in spleen macrophages. J Clin Invest 77:1776-1779

Lolait SJ, Lim ATW, Toh BH, Funder JW (1984) Immunoreactive β-endorphin in a subpopulation of mouse spleen macrophages. J Clin Invest 73:277-280

Martin J, Prystowsky MB, Angeletti RH (1987) Preproenkephalin mRNA in T-cells, macrophages and mast cells. J Neurosci Res 18:82-87

Miralles-Garcia JM, Mories-Alvarez MT, Corrales-Hernández JJ, Garcia-Diez CL (1986) β-Endorphin and male infertility. Arch Androl 16:247-251

Nappi C, Petraglia F, Cudmo V, Volpe A, Facchinetti F, Genazzani AR, Montemagno U (1989) Plasma β-endorphin levels in obese and non-obese patients with polycystic ovarian disease. Eur J Obstet Gynecol Reprod Biol 30:151-156

Piccoli R, Pasanisi A, Carsana A, Palmieri M, d'Alessio G (1988) Expression of opioid genes in bovine seminal vesicles. Eur J Biochem 172:53-58

Räisänen I (1988) Plasma levels and diurnal variation of β-endorphin, β-lipotropin and corticotropin during pregnancy and early puerperium. Eur J Obstet Gynecol Reprod Biol 27:13-20

Sibinga NES, Goldstein A (1988) Opioid peptides and opioid receptors in cells of the immune system. Annu Rev Immunol 6:219-249

Smyth DG (1983) β-Endorphin and related peptides in pituitary, brain, pancreas and antrum. Br Med Bull 39:25-30

Tepper R, Neri A, Kaufman H, Schoenfeld A, Ovadia J (1987) Menopausal hot flushes and plasma β-endorphins. Obstet Gynecol 70:150-152

Weizman A, Gil-Ad I, Grupper D, Tyano S, Laron Z (1987) The effect of acute and repeated electroconvulsive treatment on plasma β-endorphin, growth hormone, prolactin and cortisol secretion in depressed patients. Psychopharmacology (Berlin) 93:122-126

Wiedemann K, Teschemacher H (1986) Determination of β- endorphin and fragments thereof in human plasma using high-performance liquid chromatography and a multiple radioimmunoassay system. Pharmacol Res 3:142-149

Wildmann J, Krüger A, Schmole M, Niemann J, Matthaei H (1986) Increase of circulating β-endorphin-like immunoreactivity correlates with the change in feeling of pleasantness after running. Life Sci 38:997-1003

Zurawski G, Benedik M, Kamb BJ, Abrams JS, Zurawski SM, Lee FD (1986) Activation of mouse T-helper cells induces abundant preproenkephalin mRNA synthesis. Science 232:772-775

Response of Plasma Endorphins to Physical Exercise in Eumenorrheic and Amenorrheic Female Athletes[*]

T. LAATIKAINEN, H. HOHTARI, and P. RAHKILA

Introduction

It is well known that strenuous exercise may impair luteal function and cause anovulation and amenorrhea (Bullen et al.1985). The suppression of the hypo-thalamic-pituitary-ovarian (HPO) axis in exercise-associated amenorrhea is well established (Prior 1985; Ronkainen et al. 1985) but the exact cause is still unclear. Increased release of corticotropin-releasing hormone (CRH) and β-en-dorphin in the central nervous system has been proposed to be mechanisms through which stress inhibits secretion of luteinizing hormone (LH; Petraglia et al. 1986, 1987).

Cross-sectional comparisons between amenorrheic and cyclic athletes have failed to show significant differences in their exercise habits or caloric con-sumption (Drinkwater et al. 1984). Ding et al. (1988) reported that among amenorrheic athletes, those who did not have elevated serum cortisol levels spontaneously regained menstrual cycles within 6 months, while those with elevated cortisol levels remained amenorrheic. Thus the disorders of the reproductive system in women athletes may be associated with abnormalities of the hypothalamic-pituitary-adrenal (HPA) axis. It is not known whether any abnormal response of plasma endorphins or corticotropin to acute exercise is associated with disturbances of the menstrual cycle in female athletes.

Changes in the concentrations of corticotropin and β-endorphin during acute exercise reflect pituitary stress response. Many factors, e.g., intensity and duration of the exercise, training, and interindividual differences, may influence the reponse of plasma β-endorphin and corticotropin levels to exercise. The aims of this report are (a) to discuss the relationship between the intensity of exercise and the response of plasma β-endorphin and corticotropin, (b) to discuss the effect of training, and (c) to compare the response of plasma endorphins to acute exercise and to an administration of CRH in eumenorrheic and amenor-rheic athletes.

---

[*] Research supported by grants from the Academy of Finland and from the Paul Foundation, Finland.

Plasma Concentration of β-Endorphin and Corticotropin Is Dependent on a Threshold Intensity of Running Exercise in Endurance Athletes

We have studied relationships between the intensity of running exercise on a treadmill and the changes in the plasma concentrations of β-endorphin and corticotropin in ten experienced male endurance athletes (Rahkila et al. 1988). A maximum oxygen consumption (VO_{2max}) was determined for each subject using a continuous running test on a treadmill. The running speed was increased by 2 km/h at intervals of 1 min until exhaustion. At the end of the test, the mean heart rate was 185 ± 4 beats/min, the blood lactate concentration 10.1 ± 0.9 mmol/l, and VO_{2max} 65 ± 1 ml/min/kg. According to the running velocity and oxygen consumption measured during the test of maximal oxygen requirement, velocities of the treadmill were determined which would require 50%, 60%, 70%, 80%, 90%, and 100% of the individual VO_{2max}. The 50%–100% running tests were performed in a random order with an interval of 2–5 days. Blood samples were collected before and immediately after the test.

We did not find any significant change in β-endorphin and corticotropin levels in tests requiring 50%, 60%, 70%, and 80% of VO_{2max}. However, we did find a significant increase in plasma β-endorphin and corticotropin levels in response to the exercise tests requiring 90% and 100% of VO_{2max}. The increase in the plasma levels of β-endorphin and corticotropin was always accompanied by an increase of the blood lactate level. De Meirleir et al. (1986) reported that the increase in lactic acid levels above the anaerobic threshold always preceded the induced rise in β-endorphin or corticotropin levels during exercising on a bicycle ergometer. Thus, a rather high exercise rate associated with the release of lactic acid is needed to induce a rise in plasma β-endorphin or corticotropin levels in endurance athletes.

In an earlier study, we did not find any differences between male and female endurance athletes in β-endorphin or corticotropin responses to an exhaustive treadmill exercise or to a submaximal outdoor running exercise (Rahkila et al. 1987). Viswanathan et al. (1987) reported that exercise at 60% VO_{2max} level increased the plasma level of immunoreactive β-endorphin in women but not in men. Only some of the subjects in their study were trained athletes.

Effect of Training on the Basal and Exercise-Stimulated β-Endorphin Concentration

We studied the effect of training on plasma immunoreactive β-endorphin levels during acute exercise. The training group consisted of seven women with a mean age of 29.4 ± 2.0 years, mean weight 60.4 ± 1.5 kg, and mean percentage body fat $22.5 \pm 1.02\%$. The control group consisted of ten sedentary women with a mean age of 23.8 ± 0.83 years, mean weight 57.6 ± 2.03 kg, and mean percentage body fat 25.6 ± 0.85%.

The women in the training group had been practised in long-distance running or orienteering earlier, but had not been active for at least 2 months before the start of the study. The women in the control group did not participate in any training programs. The training period in the athlete group lasted for 3 months. During the 1st month the subjects ran for about 1 h 4-6 times and altogether 60-70 km a week, and after that intensified the training to 6-8 times a week to a total of 90-110 km a week. Two of the subjects with an irregular cycle became amenorrheic after the training period, one subject with a regular cycle became pregnant 1 month after the training period.

The maximum oxygen consumption (VO_{2max}) in the training group was determined for each subject at the start of the study and at the end of the 2nd and 3rd months of the training period, using a continuous running test on a treadmill to exhaustion. Then the velocities of the treadmill were determined which would require 60% and 90% of the individual VO_{2max}. Oxygen consumption was measured at 1 min intervals and blood lactate determined at the end of the test. Control subjects performed the exercise tests at the start and at the end of the study period.

Responses of plasma immunoreactive β-endorphin and corticotropin to 60% and 90% submaximal exercise were studied at intervals of 1 month in the training group and at the start and at the end of the study period in the control group. Blood samples for determinations of immunoreactive β-endorphin and corticotropin levels were collected before and immediately at the end of the 60% and 90% test. Plasma immunoreactive β-endorphin (β-endorphin + β-lipotropin) was determined by radioimmunoassay after extraction of the peptides with Sep Pak C_{18} cartriges (Laatikainen et al. 1986).

In the training group, the mean concentration of immunoreactive β-endorphin at rest was 3.8 ± 0.51 nmol/l at the start and 3.2 ± 0.34 pmol/l at the end of the training period, and the corresponding mean values of corticotropin were 2.96 ± 0.51 nmol/l and 2.19 ± 0.29 nmol/l, respectively. There was no significant difference in the mean basal values of immunoreactive β-endorphin and corticotropin before and after the training period.

A significant increase in plasma immunoreactive β-endorphin and corticotropin level was found in the 90% test but not in the 60% test. There was a highly significant correlation between the immunoreactive β-endorphin and corticotropin response to the 90% test ($r = 0.85$, $p = 0.000$), and between corticotropin and lactate values ($r = 0.60$, $p = 0.000$), and between immunoreactive β-endorphin and lactate values ($r = 0.588$, $p = 0.000$) at the end of the 90% exercise. Figure 1 shows that β-endorphin and corticotropin responses to exercise did not change during the intensive training period. No significant change was found in the control subjects in the β-endorphin and corticotropin responses during a similar time period.

We were unable to confirm the earlier reported (Carr et al. 1981) facilitation of β-endorphin response to exercise with training. The subjects studied by Carr

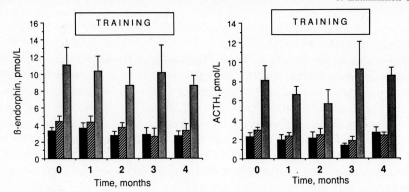

Fig. 1. Mean concentrations of immunoreactive β-endorphin and corticotropin (*ACTH*) in female endurance athletes at rest (■) and after running on a treadmill requiring 60%(▨) and 90% (▧) of maximal VO₂ before, during, and after an intensive training period.

et al. (1981) were not engaged in athletic training before the start of the study and the training period lasted for 2 months. Our findings are in accordance with those of Howlett et al. (1984), who did not find any change in β-endorphin response after an intensive training period of 8 weeks in a group of women who had not been previously used to regular exercise. Submaximal exercise tests were used in all these studies. Farrell et al. (1987) reported that in trained male subjects the response of plasma β-endorphin to very intensive (supramaximal) exercise exceeded that in untrained subjects, suggesting that chronic exposure to stress may increase the capacity of pituitary to secrete β-endorphin under very intense stress.

Plasma β-Endorphin and Corticotropin at Rest and During Physical Exercise in Eumenorrheic and Amenorrheic Female Athletes

We have studied plasma concentrations of immunoreactive β-endorphin, cortisol, and prolactin during 2 h bed rest in 9 women aged 15–18 years participating in various exercise programs and in 11 sedentary control subjects aged of 16–25 years and with regular cycles (Laatikainen et al. 1986). The blood samples were collected at 15-min intervals for 2 h, from 12.00 to 14.00 h. We found significantly increased concentrations of immunoreactive β-endorphin (3.17 ± 0.23 nmol/l vs. 2.39 ± 0.16 nmol/l, $p < 0.05$) and cortisol (274 ± 35 nmol/l vs. 134 ± 14 nmol/l, $p < 0.001$) during the 2nd h of the study (resting levels) in the group with exercise-associated amenorrhea, whereas the mean prolactin values were lower (2.4 ± 0.28 ng/l vs. 5.7 ± 1.1 ng/l, $p < 0.01$). Since neither we nor Howlett et al. (1984) were able to demonstrate any significant change in β-endorphin levels during training, this difference in immunoreactive β-endorphin levels may be related to amenorrhea rather than to training.

Villaneuva et al. (1986) found that the mean urinary 24-h cortisol levels were elevated in both amenorrheic and eumenorrheic female athletes. Recently, Loucks et al. (1989) reported that serum cortisol levels in the early morning were higher in both eumenorrheic and amenorrheic athletes in comparison to sedentary controls. This elevation lasted all the day and evening in the amenorrheic athletes. Thus, increased basal endorphin and cortisol levels suggest that the activity of the HPA axis at rest is increased in female athletes and that this change is more significant in athletes with amenorrhea.

We studied the response of plasma β-endorphin and corticotropin to a submaximal exercise in 21 healthy female endurance athletes who performed an exercise test on the bicycle ergometer, first at the level of 80% of the $VO_{2\,max}$ for 12 min, then at 100% VO_{2max} for about 2 min (Hohtari et al. 1988). Twelve of these subjects were amenorrheic and nine had regular periods. All subjects had trained regularly for an average of 6 years, weekly training activities being 12.2 ± 2.8 h in the eumenorrheic and 11.4 ± 3.6 h in the amenorrheic group. The mean weight (52.3 ± 1.9 vs. 58.6 ± 2.1 kg) and the mean percentage body fat (18.8 ± 1.4% vs. 23.4 ± 1.3%) were lower in the amenorrheic than in the eumenorrheic group.

At the end of the 80% test, the blood concentrations of lactate in the eumenorrheic and amenorrheic groups were 2.8 ± 0.33 and 3.46 ± 0.29 mmol/l, respectively, and at the end of the 100% test they were 6.98 ± 0.42 and 6.61 ± 0.38 mmol/l, respectively. There were no significant differences between the groups.

Figure 2 shows the mean concentrations of immunoreactive β-endorphin and corticotropin during the exercise. The mean percentage increase in the immunoreactive β-endorphin level was 110% in the eumenorrheic group, varying from 29% to 380%. In the amenorrheic group the responses were more variable; in two subjects no response was found and in the rest the response varied from 8.9% to 460%. Analysis of variance did not show any significant difference in immunoreactive β-endorphin or corticotropin response between the groups. There was a highly significant correlation between the increase of the immunoreactive β-endorphin and corticotropin levels during the test in the eumenorrheic ($r = 0.91$, $p < 0,001$) and the amenorrheic ($r = 0.92$, $p < 0.001$) group. The basal concentration of immunoreactive β-endorphin before the exercise was higher in the amenorrheic than in the eumenorrheic group (4.8 ± 0.8 nmol/l vs. 2.9 ± 0.2 nmol/l, $p < 0.05$). Thus, we were not able to demonstrate any significant abnormality in the response of plasma immunoreactive β-endorphin level to exercise in the amenorrheic athletes who took part in our study.

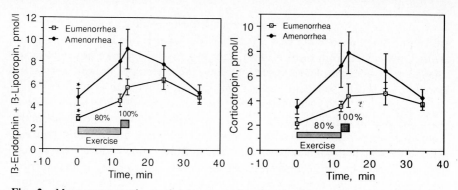

Fig. 2. Mean concentrations of immunoreactive β-endorphin and corticotropin before, during, and after acute exercise in eumenorrheic and amenorrheic athletes. (From Hohtari et al. 1988)

Response of Plasma Immunoreactive β-Endorphin and Cortisol to a CRH Test in Eumenorrheic and Amenorrheic Athletes

Pituitary response to intravenous administration of human CRH was studied in 19 female endurance athletes. Nine of them were eumenorrheic and ten amenorrheic. The clinical parameters in the eumenorrheic and amenorrheic groups respectively were as follows: age 18.7 ± 0.7 and 18.2 ± 0.46 years, weight 59.2 ± 1.7 and 51.5 ± 1.3 kg ($p = 0.003$), percentage body fat 23.5 ± 0.95 and $20.9 \pm 1.34\%$ and VO_{2max} 54.7 ± 2.27 and 62.5 ± 1.0 ml/min per kilogram ($p = 0.02$). Human CRH (Bissendorf Peptide GmbH, FRG) was administered as an intravenous bolus of 100 μg and the blood samples were collected at –15, 0, 30, 60, 90, and 120 min.

Figure 3 shows the mean changes in the plasma concentrations of immunoreactive β-endorphin and cortisol in response to the CRH test. No significant differences were found between the groups. Recently, Loucks et al. (1989) found no significant difference between amenorrheic and eumenorrheic athletes in the responses of serum corticotropin level to CRH administration, although both groups showed a blunted response in comparison to sedentary control subjects. Thus, the CRH test did not reveal any abnormality in the response of the pituitary to secrete endorphins or corticotropin in amenorrheic athletes.

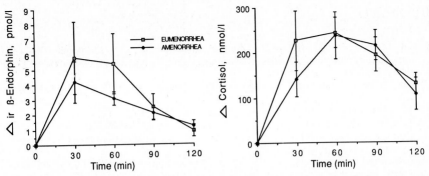

Fig. 3. Mean increase in the plasma concentrations of immunoreactive β-endorphin and cortisol after intravenous administration of a 100-μg bolus of CRH to eumenorrheic and amenorrheic athletes

Summary

In experienced athletes, strenuous exercise requiring 80%-100% of VO_{2max} increases plasma endorphin levels significantly. This was accompanied with the increase of blood lactate. There was a highly significant correlation between the response of immunoreactive β-endorphin and corticotropin level, which is explained by their common origin from the proopiomelanocortin precursor peptide.

Since training increases the VO_{2max}, this should be taken into account when the exercise intensity is expressed. When the exercise intensity was expressed as a percentage of VO_{2max} determined during the course of the training period, the responses of immunoreactive β-endorphin or corticotropin to a submaximal exercise did not change during an intensive training period. No significant changes were found in the present study in the basal immunoreactive β-endorphin or corticotropin levels during the course of the training.

We were not able to demonstrate any significant differences in the levels of plasma immunoreactive β-endorphin or corticotropin in response to exercise between eumenorrheic and amenorrheic athletes. Stimulation of pituitary β-endorphin secretion by administering a 100-μg intravenous bolus of human CRH failed to evoke any significant differences in the response of plasma immunoreactive β-endorphin between eumenorrheic and amenorrheic athletes. These studies failed to demonstrate any significant abnormalities in the pituitary response to acute stress in amenorrheic athletes.

A slightly increased basal level of immunoreactive β-endorphin was found in amenorrheic athletes. This can be related to increased plasma cortisol levels reported by other authors during the day and evening in amenorrheic athletes. These findings suggest long-term differences in response to stress between eumenorrheic and amenorrheic athletes.

References

Bullen BA, Skrinar GS, Beitins IZ, von Mering G, Turnbull BA, MacArthur JW (1985) Induction of menstrual disorders by strenous exercise in untrained women. N Engl J Med 312: 1349-1353

Carr DB, Bullen BA, Skrinar GS, Arnold MA, Rosenblatt M, Beitins IZ, Martin JB, McArthur JW (1981) Physical conditioning facilitates the exercise-induced secretion of beta-endorphin and beta lipotropin in women. N Engl J Med 305: 560-563

De Meirleir K, Naaktgeboren N, van Steirteghem A, Gorus F, Olbrecht J, Block P (1986) β-Endorphin and ACTH levels in peripheral blood during and after aerobic and anaerobic exercise. Eur J Appl Physiol 55: 5-8

Ding JH, Sheckter CB, Drinkwater BL, Soules MR, Bremner WJ (1988) High serum cortisol levels in exercise-associated amenorrhea. Ann Intern Med 108: 530-534

Drinkwater BL, Nilson K, Chesnut CH III, Bremner WJ, Shaholtz S, Southworth MB (1984) Bone mineral content of amenorrheic and eumenorrheic athletes. N Engl J Med 311: 277-281

Farrell PA, Kjaer M, Bach FW, Galbo H (1987) β-Endorphin and adrenocorticotropin response to supramaximal treadmill exercise in trained and untrained males. Acta Physiol Scand 130: 619-625

Hohtari H, Elovainio R, Salminen K, Laatikainen T (1988) Plasma corticotropin-releasing hormone, corticotropin and endorphins at rest and during exercise in eumenorrheic and amenorrheic athletes. Fertil Steril 50: 233-238

Howlett TA, Tomlin S, Ngahfoong L, Rees LH, Bullen BA, Skrinar GS, McArthur JW (1984) Release of β-endorphin and met-enkephalin during exercise in normal women: response to training. Brit Med J 288: 1950-1952

Laatikainen T, Virtanen T, Apter D (1986) Plasma immunoreactive β-endorphin in exercise-associated amenorrhea. Am J Obstet Gynecol 154: 94-97

Loucks AB, Mortola JF, Girton L, Yen SSC (1989) Alterations in the hypothalamic-pituitary-ovarian and the hypothalamic-pituitary-adrenal axes in athletic women. J Clin Endocrinol Metab 68: 402-411

Petraglia F, Sutton S, Vale W, Plotsky P (1987) Corticotropin- releasing factor decreases plasma luteinizing hormone levels in female rats by inhibiting gonadotropin-releasing hormone release into hypophyseal-portal circulation. Endocrinology 120: 1083-88

Petraglia F, Vale W, Rivier C (1986) Opioids act centrally to modulate stress-induced decrease in luteinizing hormone in the rat. Endocrinology 119: 2445-2450

Prior JC (1985) Luteal phase defects and anovulation: adaptive alterations occurring with conditioning exercise. Semin Reprod Endocrinol Metab 3: 27-33

Rahkila P, Hakala E, Alen M, Salminen K, Laatikainen T (1987) Response of plasma endorphins to running exercises in male and female endurance athletes. Med Sci Sports Exerc 19: 451-558

Rahkila P, Hakala E, Alèn M, Salminen K, Laatikainen T (1988) β-Endorphin and corticotropin release is dependent on a threshold intensity of running exercise in male endurance athletes. Life Sci 43: 551-558

Ronkainen H, Pakarinen A, Kirkinen P, Kauppila A (1985) Physical exercise-induced changes and season-associated differences in the pituitary-ovarian function of runners and joggers. J Clin Endocrinol Metab 60: 416-422

Viswanathan M, van Dijk JP, Graham TE, Bonen A, George JC (1987) Exercise-and cold-induced changes in plasma β-endorphin and β-lipotropin in men and women. J Appl Physiol 62: 622-627

Villaneuva AL, Schlosser C, Hopper B, Liu JH, Hoffman DI, Rebar Rw (1986) Increased cortisol production in women runners. J. Clin Endocrinol Metab 63: 133-136

Opioidergic Control of the Pituitary-Adrenal Axis

M. Reincke, H.M. Schulte, U. Deuss, W.Winkelmann, and B. Allolio

Introduction

Several studies in animals (Bruni et al. 1977; Rivier et al. 1977) have shown that endogenous opiate-like peptides are involved in the neuroendocrine control of pituitary hormone secretion. In man, opiates have been shown to inhibit the pituitary-adrenal axis (Grossmann 1983). Thus, β-endorphin suppresses basal ACTH and cortisol secretion (Taylor et al. 1983). Similarly, the δ-opiate receptor agonist morphine sulfate reduces baseline cortisol concentrations (McDonald et al. 1959) and blocks the cortisol response to surgical stress (George et al. 1974; Brandt et al. 1978). The met-enkephalin analog FK 33-824, a synthetic derivative acting at u-and δ-opiate receptor sites (Kream and Zukin 1979) completely blocks the ACTH response to lysine-vasopressin (del Pozo et al. 1980). Recently it has been reported that the racemic benzomorphan κ-agonist MR 2033 also decreases ACTH and cortisol secretion (Pfeiffer et al. 1986). Thus, there is evidence that the inhibitory action of opiates on the pituitary-adrenal axis involves u-, δ-, and κ-binding sites. However, the physiological role and the site of action of endogenous and exogenous opioids remain to be elucidated. In recent years we have therefore studied the effect of FK 33-824, oral morphine, and naloxone on baseline and releasing hormone-stimulated ACTH and cortisol concentrations in patients with Addison's disease and normal subjects.

Effect of Met-Enkephalin Analog on ACTH Secretion in Patients with Addison's Disease

Seven patients with Addison's disease were studied. All tests were performed at 09.00 h, after an overnight fast. Substitution therapy was withheld for at least 16 h before the tests. The patients were studied on four occasions in a cross over study; they received:

1. 0.5 mg FK 33-824, a long-acting analog of met-enkephalin (Sandoz Ltd., Basel, Switzerland), i.m. or
2. Placebo (0.9% saline i.m.) or
3. 4 mg naloxone (Narcanti, Du Pont, Frankfurt, FRG) i.v. or
4. 4 mg naloxone i.v. and 0.5 mg FK 33-824 i.m.

Naloxone was administered as a bolus injection 5 min before the enkephalin injection. Blood samples for ACTH determinations were drawn at frequent intervals.

Written informed consent was obtained from all subjects in this and the following studies. The hormone measurements of this and the other protocols were performed as follows: plasma ACTH and plasma immunoreactive (ir)-β-endorphin were determined by radioimmunoassay after extraction from plasma (Voigt et al. 1974) as described previously (Jeffcoate et al. 1978; Allolio et al. 1981). The antibody against β-endorphin showed 28% crossreactivity with β-lipotropin on a molar basis. We used synthetic β-endorphin (Universal Biologicals, Cambridge, UK) for iodination and standard. Cortisol was measured by radioimmunoassay using commercially available reagents (Du Pont, New England Nuclear, Dreieich, FRG).

Statistical evaluation was performed using the Student's paired t test and the Wilcoxon nonparametric test for paired data. All values are expressed as mean ± SEM.

In all patients with Addison's disease, FK 33-824 consistently produced a rapid striking fall of plasma ACTH levels (Fig. 1). The suppression of plasma ACTH levels, expressed as a percentage of the basal samples, reached a nadir at 120 min (mean ± SEM, $p < 0.001$ compared to placebo).

Naloxone provoked a significant rise of plasma ACTH in patients with Addison's disease ($p < 0.005$). After 1 h, ACTH concentrations had returned to the placebo levels. The administration of FK 33-824 together with naloxone alone produced a decrease in ACTH ($p < 0.01$) which was significantly less substantial than the decrease observed when FK 33-824 was administered alone.

Effect of Met-Enkephalin Analog on CRH-Stimulated Hormone Levels in Normal Subjects

Seven healthy volunteers participated in this study. On two occasions all subjects underwent a CRF test (0.1 mg human CRH i.v., Bachem Inc., Bubendorf, Switzerland). In random order the two tests were combined with administration of either FK 33-824 (0.5 mg i.m.) or placebo (0.9% saline i.m.) 60 min prior to the hCRH injection. Blood samples for ACTH, ir-β-endorphin and cortisol were collected at frequent intervals.

In all subjects hCRH elicited an increase in plasma ACTH and ir-β-endorphin, which was paralleled by a rise in serum cortisol. This increase was almost completely blocked by prior administration of FK 33-824 (Fig. 2). After FK 33-824, peak ACTH concentrations in response to hCRH were reduced from 45.3 ± 7.8 to 16.7 ± 3.5 pg/ml ($p > 0.02$). The same held true for plasma ir-β-endorphin concentrations and for serum cortisol levels ($p < 0.02$).

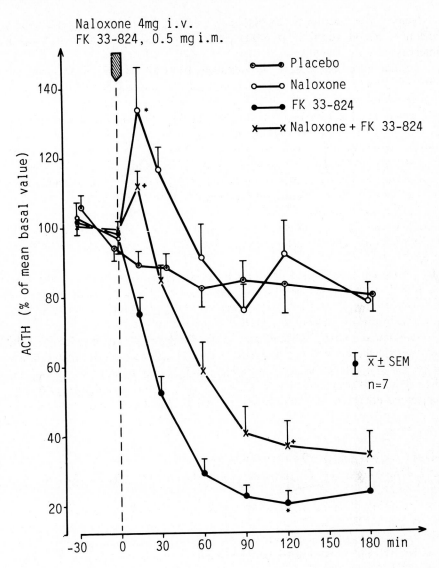

Fig. 1. Plasma ACTH (mean percentage variations) in patients with Addison's disease after administration of FK 33-824 (0.5 mg i.m.), placebo (0.9% saline i.m.), naloxone (4 mg i.v.), or naloxone + FK 33-824. Naloxone was given as a bolus injection 5 min before FK 33-824

Effect of Naloxone on Plasma ACTH in Addison's Disease

Seven patients suffering from primary adrenal insufficiency were studied. All tests were started at 08.30 h after an overnight fast. Substitution therapy was

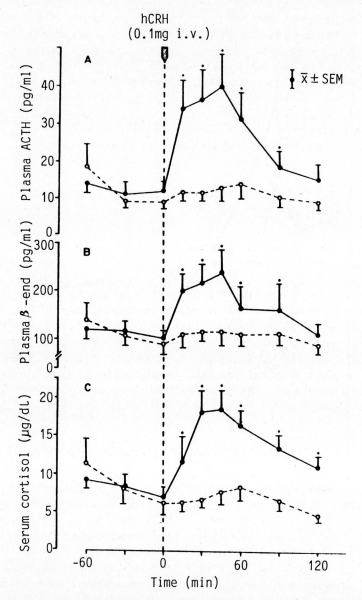

Fig. 2A-C. Effect of FK 33-824 (○——○) vs. placebo (●——●) on hCRH-induced increase in plasma ACTH, plasma ir-β-endorphin, and serum cortisol in normal subjects. * $p < 0.02$

withheld for at least 24 h before the tests. Using a double blind crossover protocol all patients received placebo (0.9% saline), a low-dose infusion of naloxone (0.8 mg/h) and a high-dose infusion of naloxone (5.4 mg/h) i.v. over a period of 90 min, with blood sampling at 15, 30, 60, 90, and 120 min.

In all patients the infusion of high-dose naloxone resulted in a significant increase in plasma ACTH concentrations lasting throughout the time of naloxone infusion. Maximum plasma ACTH levels were $165 \pm 25\%$ versus $82 \pm 6\%$ (percentage of basal values; $p < 0.02$ compared to placebo). In contrast, plasma ACTH levels were unaffected by infusion of low-dose naloxone.

Effect of Naloxone on Pituitary-Adrenal Response in Man Induced by hCRH

On two occasions 13 healthy volunteers underwent a hCRH test (0.1 mg i.v.). After an overnight fast, seven volunteers received 4 mg nalaxone or placebo (0.9% saline) as an intravenous bolus injection at 10.55 h followed by hCRH at 11.00 h. Six volunteers received 4 mg naloxone as an intravenous bolus injection at 16.55 h, followed by a continuous infusion of 6 mg of naloxone over 75 min or placebo (0.9% saline). hCRH was injected at 17.00 h. Blood sampled for measuring cortisol, ACTH, and ir-β-endorphin were collected.

Administration of 4 mg naloxone as a bolus dose at -5 min did not alter the hormone response to hCRH. In contrast, compared with placebo, high-dose naloxone (10 mg) significantly enhanced the hormone release after hCRH (Fig.3; $p < 0.05$).

Effect of Oral Morphine on Pituitary-Adrenal Axis in Man

On two occasions seven normal subjects underwent a hCRH test (0.1 mg i.v.). After an overnight fast, the volunteers received 30 mg of a slow-release morphine sulfate preparation (1 tablet MST 30, Mundipharma, Limburg, FRG) or placebo at 08.00 h. At 11.00 h the hCRH test was performed.

Compared with placebo, administration of oral morphine resulted in a significant ($p < 0.002$) suppression of basal serum cortisol, plasma ACTH, and plasma ir-β-endorphin at 180 min. In addition, peak hormone values in response to hCRH were significantly reduced ($p < 0.02$; Fig. 4)

Discussion

Our data show that in Addison's disease FK 33-824 induced a long- lasting suppression of plasma ACTH, reaching levels below 25% of baseline values. This effect was partly reversed by 4 mg naloxone. These results demonstrate

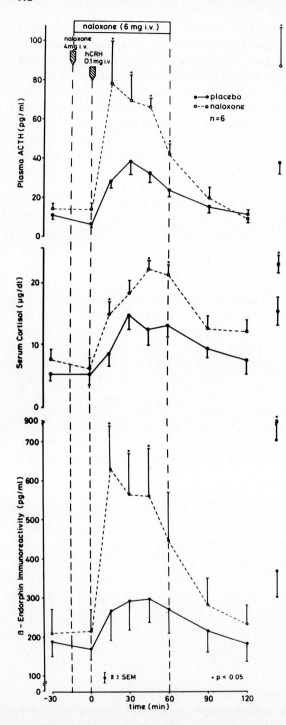

Fig. 3. Plasma ACTH, serum cortisol, and plasma ir-β-endorphin concentrations after hCRH administration (0.1 mg i.v. at 0 min) in six subjects after placebo (0.9% saline) (●——●) and after the same stimulus plus naloxone (4 mg i.v. at -15 min followed by infusion of 6 mg over 75 min; ○——○). Maximum hormone concentrations are depicted on the right

that in patients with Addison's disease ACTH release is influenced by inhibitory opiate receptors which are relatively naloxone-resistant. Furthermore, inhibition of the endogenous opiate action by competitive blockade of the receptors with 8 mg naloxone (i.v. over 90 min), but not with low-dose naloxone (1.2 mg i.v. over 90 min) induced an elevation of plasma ACTH levels. This indicates that ACTH secretion is tonically inhibited by endogenous opiate peptides, probably mediated by relatively naloxone-insensitive δ-or κ-receptors.

These results are in agreement with previous studies. Gaillard et al. (1981) found a similar ACTH decrease in response to intravenous FK 33-284 injections in patients with Addison's disease. The suppression of plasma ACTH was completely reversed by prior administration of 8 mg naloxone. In normal subjects a 10 mg dose of naloxone has been shown to increase secretion of ACTH and cortisol (Morley et al. 1980), whereas 4 mg naloxone as a bolus were ineffective to raise serum cortisol levels (del Pozo et al. 1980). In addition, in our study high-dose but not low-dose naloxone increased the hormonal response to hCRH in normal subjects. These results allow the assumption of dose-dependent effects of naloxone, via less naloxone-sensitive δ-or κ- receptors, on ACTH secretion. Our studies with the μ-and δ-agonist FK 33-824 strongly suggest a role of δ-opiate receptors, as only high doses of naloxone reverse its effects on the pituitary-adrenal axis.

Since endogenous opiates play an important inhibitory role in controlling ACTH secretion, this inhibition may be responsible for the circadian rhythm of the pituitary-adrenal axis. However, Grossmann et al. (1982) demonstrated that high-dose naloxone administered to normal subjects led to a constant rise in plasma ACTH and serum cortisol concentrations, irrespective of the time of administration (9.00 h, 18.00 h, and 23.00 h). This suggests that the pituitary-adrenal axis is under constant tonic inhibition by endogenous peptides throughtout the 24 h, and that endogenous peptides are not involved in circadian ACTH secretion.

In normal subjects we found a pronounced inhibition of the CRH-induced ACTH and β-endorphin release by FK 33-284. These data support the concept of a direct effect of this opioid at the pituitary level, although additional suprahypophyseal sites cannot be excluded. Since high concentrations of endogenous opioids have been demonstrated in the hypothalamus (Watson et al. 1978) as well as in the pituitary gland (Gramsch et al. 1978), opioids may act in an inhibitory manner at either site.

In normal subjects we observed incomplete suppression of the hCRH-induced ACTH, β-endorphin, and cortisol release by oral morphine sulfate. These data provide evidence for the involvement of δ-opiate receptors in the opioidergic control of ACTH secretion, since morphine sulfate is known to be a pure μ-receptor agonist. Furthermore, because the suppression of ACTH release was incomplete, morphine sulfate probably acts at the level of the hypothalamus.

So far, only inhibitory actions of endogenous and exogenous opiates on ACTH secretion in man have been observed (Grossmann and Clement-Jones (1983). Our data and previous studies support the concept of a continuous

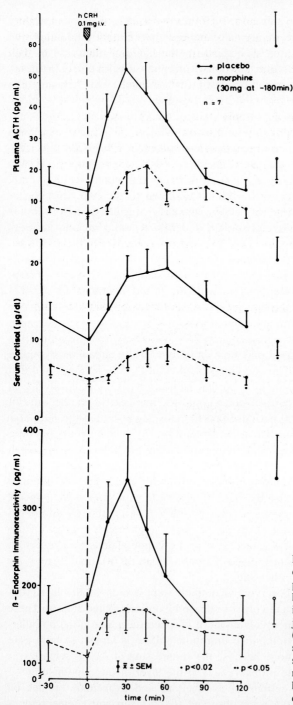

Fig. 4. Plasma ACTH, serum cortisol and plasma ir-β-endorphin concentrations after hCRH administration (0.1 mg i.v. at 0 min) in seven subjects after placebo (●——●) and after the same stimulus plus morphine sulfate (30 mg orally at -180 min; ○——○). Maximum hormone concentrations are depicted on the right

inhibitory tone exerted by opiates on the pituitary-adrenal axis day and night. Hormone secretion from the pituitary corticotroph is probably modulated by local met-enkephalin or β-endorphin acting in the hypothalamus and in the pituitary. Our data show that μ-and δ-opiate receptors are involved in these actions. Pfeiffer et al. (1986) demonstrated that κ-opiate receptors too are involved in the inhibitory control of ACTH secretion.

Endogenous opiate peptides probably induce a suppression of endogenous CRH and of CRH costimulating factors like catecholamines, vasopressin, and angiotensin II at the level of the hypothalamus, which in turn inhibits ACTH release (Fig. 5, Ia). Our results suggest, in addition to the suprahypophyseal site of action, a direct effect of opiates at the level of the pituitary corticotoph (Fig.5, Ib). However, this concept is controversial (Grossmann et al. 1986). An alternative explanation for the inhibitory action of opiates may be a hypothetical ACTH-suppressing factor (Fig. 5, II). In this concept, endogenous opiates stimulate secretion of a hypothalamic factor, which exerts its inhibitory effects via the portal vessels on the corticotoph.

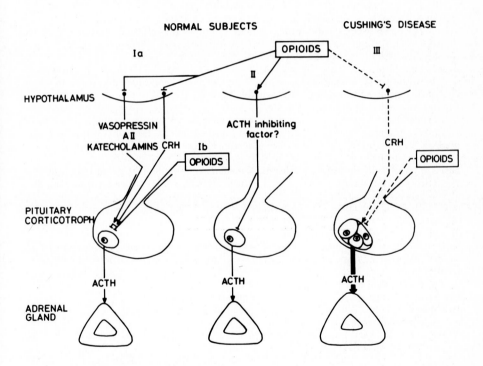

Fig. 5. The opioidergic control of the pituitary adrenal axis (for details see text). *A II*, angiotensin II; ————> stimulatory action; ————⊣, inhibitory action

In patients with pituitary-dependent Cushing's disease we demonstrated that ACTH hypersecretion is insensitive to FK 33-824 and to naloxone (Allolio et al. 1982; Deuß et al. 1985). Furthermore, in contrast to normal subjects, the hCRH-induced ACTH increase in these patients was not blocked by prior administration of FK 33-824 (Allolio et al. 1986). These data point to a defect in the opioidergic control of ACTH secretion in patients with Cushing's disease (Fig. 5, III).

Acknowledgements, We are indebted to Miss D. Vollmar, Mrs. H. Hofmann, Miss M. Krietemeyer, and Mrs. G. Rossbach for skillful technical assistance.

References

Allolio B, Winkelmann W, Hipp FX (1981) Effect of meclastine, an H_1 antihistamine, on plasma ACTH in adrenal insufficiency. Acta Endocrinol (Copenh) 96:98-102

Allolio B, Winkelmann W, Hipp FX, Kaulen D, Mies R, (1982) Effects of a met-enkephalin analog on adrenocorticotropin (ACTH), growth hormone, and prolactin in patients with ACTH hypersecretion. J Clin Endocrinol Metab 55:1-7

Allolio B, Deuss U, Kaulen D, Leonhardt U, Kallabis D, Hamel E, Kaufmann W (1986) FK 33-284, a met-enkephalin analog, blocks corticotropin-releasing hormone induced adrenocorticotropin secretion in normal subjects but not in patients with Cushing's disease. J Clin Endocrinol Metab 63:1427-1431

Brandt MR, Korshin J, Prange Hansen A, Hunner L, Nistrup Madsen S, Rugg I, Kehlet H (1978) Influence of morphine anaesthesia on the endocrine metabolic response to open-heart surgery. Acta Anaesthesiol Scand 22:400-412

Bruni J, van Vogt D, Marshall S, Meites J (1977) Effects of naloxone, morphine and methionine enkephalin on serum prolactin, luteinizing hormone, follicle stimulating hormone, thyroid stimulating hormone and growth hormone. Life Sci 21:461-463

del Pozo E, von Graffenried B, Brownell J, Derrer F, Marbach P (1980) Endocrine effect of a met-enkephalin derivative (FK 33-824) in man. Horm Res 13:90-97

Deuss U, Allolio B, Kaulen D, Fischer H, Winkelmann W (1985) Effects of high-dose and low-dose naloxone on plasma ACTH in patients with ACTH hypersecretion. Clin Endocrinol (Oxf) 22:273-279

Gaillard RC, Grossmann A, Smith R, Rees LH, Besser GM (1981) The effects of a met-enkephalin analogue on ACTH, β-LPH, β-endorphin and met-enkephalin in patients with adrenocortical disease. Clin Endocrinol (Oxf) 14:471-478

George JM, Reier CE, Lanese RR, Power JM (1974) Morphine anesthesia blocks cortisol and growth hormone response to surgical stress in humans. J Clin Endocrinol 38:735-741

Gramsch C, Höllt V, Mehraein P, Pasi A, Herz A (1978) Regional distribution of endorphins in human brain and pituitary. JN: Van Ree JM, Teremins L (Eds): Characteristics and function of opioids. Elsevier/North Holland, Amsterdam, 277-281.

Grossmann A, et al. (1982) Opiate modulation of the pituitary- adrenal axis: effects of stress and circadian rhythm. Clin Endocrinol (Oxf) 17:279-286

Grossmann A and Clement-Jones V. (1983) Brain opiates and neuroendocrine function. Clin Endocrinol Metab 12:725-746

Grossmann A, et al. (1986) An analogue of met-enkephalin atenuates the pituitary-adrenal response to ovine corticotrophin releasing factor. Clin Endocrinol (Oxf) 25:421-426

Jeffcoate WJ, Rees LH, Lowry PJ, Besser GM (1978) A specific radioimmunoassy for human β-lipotropin. J Clin Endocrinol Metab 47:160-167

Kream RM, Zukin S (1979) Binding characteristics of a potent enkephalin analogue. Biochem Biophys Res Commun 90:99-109

McDonald RK, Evans FT, Weise VK, Patrick RW (1959) Effect of morphine and nalorphine on plasma hydrocortisone levels in man. J Pharmacol Exp Ther 125:241-247

Morley JE, Baranetsky NG, Wingert TD, Carlson HE, Hershman JM, Melmed S, Levin SR, Jannison KR, Weitzmann R, Chang RJ, Varner AA (1980) Endocrine effects of naloxone-induced opiate receptor blockade. J Clin Endocrinal Metab 50:251-254

Pfeiffer A, Knepel W, Braun S, Meyer HD, Lohmann H, Brantl V (1986) Effects of a kappa-opioid agonist on adrenocorticotropic and diuretic function in man. Horm Metab Res 18:842-848

Rivier C, Vale W, Ling N, Brown M, Guillemin R (1977) Stimulation in vivo of the secretion of prolactin and growth hormone by β-endorphin. Endocrinology 100:238-241

Taylor T, Dluhy RG, Williams GH (1983) β-Endorphin suppresses adrenocorticotropin and cortisol levels in normal human subjects. J Clin Endocrinol Metab 57:592-597

Voigt KH, Fehm HE, Reck R, Pfeiffer EF (1974) Spontaneous and stimulated secretion of QUSO-extractable immunoassayable ACTH in man. Klin Wochenschr 52:516-521

Watson SJ, Akil H, Richard CW, Barches JD (1978) Evidence for two separate opiate peptide neuronal systems. Nature 275:226-228

Effects of β-Endorphin on Adrenocortical Steroid Secretion

K.SZ. Szalay

For a long period adrenocorticotropin (ACTH) was thought to be the only hormone responsible for adrenocortical steroid secretion. However, it eventually became evident (Mains et al. 1977) that ACTH is synthesized in the pituitary as part of a large precursor glycoprotein, named proopiomelanocortin by Chretien et al. (1979). This precursor also contains β-LPH, γ-LPH, β-endorphin (β-EP), met-enkephalin, and α-, β-, and γ-melanocyte-stimulating hormone (MSH; Eipper and Mains 1980) which are cosecreted with ACTH.

A series of studies has been carried out to investigate the roles of these peptides in the regulation of adrenocortical steroid secretion. This paper concentrates on the effects of β-EP, reviews the literature, summarizes the results of our earlier studies, and presents our new results in this field.

Immunoreactive β-EP has been detected in human plasma (Nakao et al. 1978) and has been shown to be secreted from the hypophysis concomitantly with ACTH and other peptide fragments of proopiomelanocortin in response to a variety of stimuli (Nakao et al. 1978, 1979; Wiedemann et al. 1979). Adrenalectomy elevates and dexamethasone administration reduces the concentrations of both ACTH and β-EP in plasma (Guillemin et al. 1977). Both β-EP and ACTH synthesis are under the negative regulatory control of glucocorticoids in AtT-20 cells (Vale et al. 1978). This parallelism in the regulation of ACTH and β-EP stimulated many research groups to examine the role of β-EP in the regulation of adrenocortical glucocorticoid synthesis.

Another intriguing question was the role of β-EP in the regulation of aldosterone secretion, as it has long been suspected that, besides ACTH, another pituitary hormone also plays a role in the regulation of aldosterone secretion (Szalay 1981). Numerous studies attempted to find this hormone in various parts of proopiomelanocortin, and β-endorphin was one of the candidates as the so far unidentified pituitary aldosteronotropic factor.

To investigate the effects of β-EP on adrenocortical steroidogenesis, we used collagenase-digested adrenal capsular strippings to yield a preparation of zona glomerulosa cells, and of decapsulated adrenal gland to yield zona fasciculata cells (Szalay and Stark 1981). Synthetic human β-EP was added to the cell suspensions in concentrations of $10^{-12} - 10^4$ M alone or together with 1.6×10^{-10} M α_h^{1-39}ACTH. $10^{-11} - 10^{-5}$ M β-EP decreased, whereas 5×10^{-5} and 10^{-4} M β-EP increased the corticosterone production of zona fasciculata cells ($p < 0.01$ at $10^{-11} - 10^{-9}$, 5×10^{-5} and 10^{-4} M, Fig. 1.) $10^{-12} - 5 \times 10^{-5}$

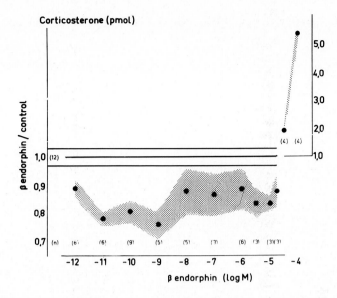

Fig. 1. Effect of β-endorphin on the corticosterone production of zona fasciculata cells. *Stippled area*, range of SEM. (Mean ± SEM. basal production of corticosterone was 105.9 ± 9.1 pmol/ml, $n = 12$)

M β-EP did not affect the steroid production of zona glomerulosa cells, but 10^{-4} M β-EP increased both their corticosterone and aldosterone production (Table 1).

The stimulatory effect of ACTH on zona fasciculata corticosterone production was decreased by $10^{-9} - 10^{-7}$ M β-EP ($p < 0.01$, Fig. 2). β-EP decreased the aldosterone production stimulated by ACTH, but did not affect glomerulosa corticosterone production (Table 2).

10^{-6} M naloxone failed to influence the reducing effect of β-EP on zona fasciculata corticosterone production (Table 3).

Our results indicated that β-EP in concentrations that may be considered physiological inhibited both basal and ACTH-stimulated corticosterone synthesis in zona fasciculata cells and inhibited basal aldosterone synthesis in zona glomerulosa cells.

A review of the literature reveals three possibilities as regards the effects of β-EP on adrenocortical steroid synthesis: inhibitory (similarly to our results in low doses), stimulatory (similarly to our results in high doses), and no effect at all (similarly to the results of some of our recent experiments, which will be presented below). This is true for both glucocorticoid and aldosterone production. I shall summarize the various results and attempt to explain the different effects of β-EP on adrenocortical steroid synthesis.

Table 1. Effect of β-endorphin on aldosterone and corticosterone production of zona glomerulosa cells (values shown are the ratios of stimulated and control cell suspensions, mean ± SEM)

	None	10^{-12}	10^{-11}	10^{-10}	10^{-9}	10^{-8}	10^{-7}	10^{-6}	5×10^{-6}	10^{-5}	2.5×10^{-5}	5×10^{-5}	10^{-4}
						β-Endophorin (M)							
Ald.	1.00 ± 0.047	0.96 ± 0.045	0.96 ± 0.042	1.01 ± 0.029	1.00 ± 0.016	1.06 ± 0.024	1.01 ± 0.056	1.00 ± 0.032	0.90 ± 0.020	1.01 ± 0.017	1.04 ± 0.076	1.08 ± 0.039	1.31 ± 0.063
B	1.00 ± 0.029	0.87 ± 0.082	0.93 ± 0.028	0.95 ± 0.052	0.95 ± 0.035	1.00 ± 0.028	1.09 ± 0.040	0.92 ± 0.060	0.95 ± 0.046	0.95 ± 0.047	1.00 ± 0.047	1.13 ± 0.042	1.47** ± 0.075
	(11)	(5)	(6)	(9)	(5)	(6)	(3)	(6)	(3)	(3)	(3)	(3)	(3)

Ald., aldosterone;   B, Coricosterone;   (n); $p < 0.01$

Table 2. Effect of β-endorphin on the zona glomerulosa steroid secreting stimulating activity of 1.6×10^{-10} ACTH (values shown are the ratios of ACTH + β-endorphin treated and ACTH treated cell suspensions, mean ± SEM)

	None	10^{-12}	10^{-11}	10^{-10}	10^{-9}	10^{-8}	10^{-7}	10^{-6}	10^{-5}	2.5×10^{-5}
						β-Endorphin(M)				
Ald.	1.00 ± 0.027	0.93 ± 0.060	0.92 ± 0.039	0.94 ± 0.032	0.83* ± 0.039	0.88 ± 0.044	0.74** ± 0.022	0.85 ± 0.050	0.97 ± 0.053	1.05 ± 0.055
B	1.00 ± 0.012	1.02 ± 0.057	0.98 ± 0.026	0.97 ± 0.017	0.99 ± 0.024	1.02 ± 0.029	1.00 ± 0.034	0.97 ± 0.013	1.07 ± 0.028	1.13 ± 0.046
	(21)	(6)	(6)	(9)	(6)	(6)	(3)	(6)	(3)	(3)

Ald., aldosterone;   B, coricosterone;   (n);   * $p < 0.05$ ** $p < 0.01$

Mean ± SEM basal production of aldosterone was 2.65 ± 0.31 pmol/ml ($n = 11$)

mean ± SEM of the ACTH-stimulated aldosterone was 57.8 ± 5.99 pmol/ml ($n = 21$).

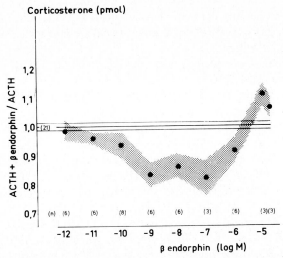

Fig. 2. Effect of β-endorphin on the zona fasciculata corticosterone secretion stimulating activity of 1.6×10^{-10} ACTH. *Stippled area*, range of SEM. (Mean ± SEM. basal production of corticosterone was 105.9 ± 9.1 pmol/ml, $n = 12$; mean ± SEM of ACTH stimulated corticosterone was 2981.2 ± 169.2 pmol/ml, $n = 21$)

Table 3. Effect of β-endorphin and naloxone on zona fasciculata corticosterone production (pmol/ml, mean ± SEM, $n = 6$)

	Corticosterone produced	
	− Naloxone	+ Naloxone, $10^{-6}\,M$
Control	75.4 ± 2.05	76.6 ± 2.39
β-EP $10^{-10}\,M$	55.1 ± 4.77*	50.3 ± 4.13
β-EP $10^{-9}\,M$	52.9 ± 2.37*	52.6 ± 1.50
β-EP $10^{-8}\,M$	62.2 ± 2.40*	61.0 ± 3.58

* $p < 0.05$

Most authors claim that β-EP has no direct effect on corticosteroidogenesis. However, in some of these studies only one dose is used (Lamberts et al. 1983; Pham-Huu-Trung et al. 1982), or the data are not shown (Matsuoka et al. 1980; Pham-Huu-Trung et al. 1985; Washburn et al. 1982). There are papers stating that β-EP has no effect, but the data presented clearly demonstrate an inhibitory effect; for example in Fig. 3 of the paper of Matsuoka et al. (1981), $10^{-9} - 5 \times 10^{-5}\,M$ β-EP inhibits the corticosterone production of decapsulated rat adrenal cells. The same is true for the study by Güllner and Gill (1983), who infused 3 pmol/min β-EP for 50 min into hypophysectomized, nephrectomized dogs. They reported that aldosterone secretion was increased and "cortisol secretion was not affected," but in Fig. 1 a distinct difference can be seen: in dogs infused with β-EP, the cortisol secretion was lower than in those infused with normal saline.

The most convincing data about the ineffectivity of β-EP towards steroidogenesis are those of Goverde et al. (1988): $1.5 \times 10^{-11} - 1.5 \times 10^{-6} M$ β-EP had no effect on either the basal or the ACTH-stimulated corticosterone production of purified isolated rat adrenal cells.

On the other hand, there are two studies that seem to prove the inhibitory effect of β-EP. Taylor et al. (1983) infused β-EP (0.3, 1.0, and 3.0 ng/kg. min, each dose for 30 min) into normal subjects. These doses of β-EP significantly suppressed the ACTH and cortisol levels. The decline in ACTH level was less consistent than the suppression of cortisol, which also shows the possibility of a direct inhibitory effect of β-EP. In the experiments of Beyer et al. (1986), the integrated cortisol response to exogenous ACTH (calculated as the area under the cortisol response curve) was significantly less when the ACTH infusion was preceded by a 30-min β-EP infusion than when ACTH was administered alone to dexamethasone-pretreated human subjects.

The third type of studies argues for the stimulatory effect of β-EP on glucocorticoid secretion. Shanker and Sharma (1979) found that β-EP stimulated the corticosterone production of trypsin-digested isolated rat adrenocortical cells in a sigmoid concentration–response manner: the maximum increase resulted at $10^{-7} M$. The effects of ACTH and β-EP were not additive.

In the experiments of Guaza et al. (1986) $10^{-10} - 10^{-6} M$ β-EP increased the basal corticosteroidogenesis and also the adrenal response to a submaximally effective dose of ACTH. The influence of β-EP upon the basal steroidogenesis exhibited an inverted U-shaped dose–response relationship; on increase of the dose to $10^{-4} M$, the stimulatory effect was reduced.

Eggens et al. (1987) reported that 10^{-6} β-EP stimulated the secretion of cortisol by isolated human adrenocortical cells.

As concerns the role of β-EP in the regulation of aldosterone production, the most interesting contradictory results are to be found in one particular issue of the *Journal of Clinical Endocrinology*. In the studies by Rabinowe et al. (1985), normal human subjects received a human synthetic β-EP infusion in successive doses of 0.3, 1.0, and 3.0 µg/kg. min for 30 min each. The plasma cortisol level fell, while both the plasma renin activity and the plasma aldosterone level were increased. After termination of the 90-min β-EP infusion, the plasma renin activity gradually returned toward the basal level, while the plasma aldosterone remained elevated for an additional 120 min. It was concluded that β-EP stimulates aldosterone release in vivo; an early aldosterone rise may be secondary to an increase in renin release, but there must be an additional direct or indirect effect of β-EP on aldosterone secretion. However, the opposite result was found by Kem et al. (1985). Synthetic human β-EP was infused into normal subjects at a dosage level several orders of magnitude higher than the endogenous levels. No increase in plasma aldosterone was found in these subjects, despite the fact that other biological actions (significant responses of pancreatic glucagon and insulin) of β-EP were manifested.

It is beyond the scope of this short review to deal with the effects of the other endogenous opiate met-enkephalin on adrenocortical steroid secretion. However, it should be mentioned that, as for β-EP, there are contradictory data about its effects in the literature. Some of the data point to a direct inhibitory effect of met-enkephalin (Ràcz et al. 1980), whereas others suggest that met-enkephalin has not direct effect at the adrenocortical level (Lamberts et al. 1983). The stimulatory effect of met-enkephalin on adrenocortical steroid secretion is indirect; it seems to be a consequence of the increase in ACTH secretion (de Souza and van Loon 1982).

To summarize, there are three types of response of adrenocortical corticosteroid synthesis to β-EP, and it is natural that everybody believes in his/her own data and tries to explain the contradictory results in terms of methodological and species differences. Let us face the facts: the experiments cited above all reflect the truth. The action of β-EP on adrenocortical steroid synthesis is sometimes inhibitory and sometimes stimulatory, but in most cases it is ineffective.

I have attempted to establish the cause of the differences in the responses of adrenocortical cells to β-EP, which could well be a reflection of the different functional states of the adrenocortical cells. To test this hypothesis, I have repeated the experiments described earlier (Szalay and Stark 1981) and presented again here, on dexamethasone-and ACTH-pretreated rats.

Rats were treated with 1 mg/kg dexamethasone (Oradexon, Organon) i.p. 4 h before decapitation or with 200 µg/kg ACTH (Synacthen Depot, CIBA.) i.m. 2 h before decapitation. Controls were injected with physiological saline i.p. 4 h before decapitation. Cell separation and incubation were carried out as described above. This time β-EP inhibited zona fasciculata corticosterone production only in dexamethasone-pretreated rats (Fig. 3, D, $p < 0.05$ at $10^{-8}M$ $p < 0.01$ at $10^{-7}M$). Aldosterone production was inhibited by β-EP in dexamethasone-pretreated rats (Fig. 4, D, $p < 0.05$ at 10^{-9} M) and stimulated in ACTH-pretreated animals (Fig. 4, A, $p < 0.05$ at 10^{-8} M).

These results show that the different effects of β-EP can be partly explained by the previous state (hypo-or hyperfunction) of the adrenocortical cells.

My hypothesis for the mechanism of the different β-EP effects is as follows: it is possible that β-EP may bind to opioid as well as to ACTH receptors in the adrenocortical cells. If it binds to opioid receptors, adenylcyclase is inhibited (Giagnoni et al. 1977), and thus steroid secretion is inhibited too. If it binds to ACTH receptors, adenylcyclase is stimulated, and thus steroid secretion is stimulated too. How β-EP acts on steroidogenesis depends on the proportions of opiate and ACTH receptor binding. Whether β-EP is bound to opioid or ACTH receptors may depend on various experimental circumstances, such as ionic concentrations, pH, temperature, and the previous occupancy of the receptors. For example, one of the most characteristic features of opiate receptor binding in the brain is its selective alteration by Na^+ (Simantov and Snydes

Zona fasciculata corticosterone

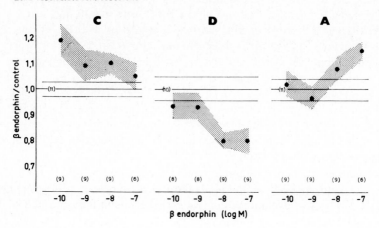

Fig. 3. Effect of β-endorphin on the corticosterone production of zona fasciculata cells of rats treated with *C* physiological saline or *D* 1 mg/kg dexamethasone i.p. 4 h before, or *A* 200 μg/kg ACTH i.m. 2 h before decapitation. (Mean ± SEM basal production of corticosterone was C 133 ± 10, D 151± 19, A 142 ± 16 pmol/ml)

Zona glomerulosa aldosterone

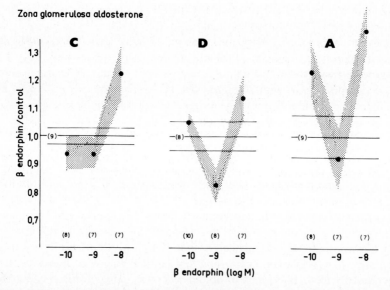

Fig. 4. Effect of β-endorphin on the aldosterone production of zona glomerulosa cells of rats treated with *C* physiological saline, or *D* 1 mg/kg dexamethasone i.p. 4 h before, or *A* 200 μg/kg ACTH i.m. 2 h before decapitation. (Mean ± SEM basal production of aldosterone was *C* 1702 ± 93, *D* 2281 ± 263, *A* 1209 ± 153 pmol/ml)

1977). In the experiments of Gibson et al. (1979), the effects of opioid agonists and antagonists on ACTH-induced steroidogenesis were dependent on the concentration of sodium in the medium. The binding of β-EP most probably depends on the Ca^{2+} concentration too. Rácz et al. (1980) reported that the inhibitory action of enkephalins on corticosteroid synthesis could be augmented by increasing the Ca^{2+} concentration in the cell-containing medium.

To summarize: according to our present knowledge, β-EP may modify adrenocortical steroid synthesis, its effect depending on the actual local *milieu interieur*. Only carefully planned studies to measure the binding of β-EP to adrenocortical cells, together with its effect on corticosteroidogenesis, can reveal the physiological role of β-EP in adrenocortical steroid synthesis.

References

Beyer HM, Parker L, Li CH, Stuart D, Sharp BM (1986) β- Endorphin attenuates the serum cortisol response to exogenous adrenocorticotropin. J Clin Endocrinol Metab 62:808-811

Chretien M, Benjannet S, Gossard F, Gianoulakis C, Crine P, Lis M, Seidah NG (1979) From β-lipotropin to β-endorphin and pro-opiomelanocortin. Can J Biochem 57:1111-1121

De Souza EB, van Loon GR (1982) D-ala^2-met-enkephalinamide, a potent opioid peptide, alters pituitary-adrenocortical secretion in rats. Endocrinology 111:1483-1490

Diel F, Holz J, Bethge N (1981) Failure of somatostatin and β-endorphin to affect bovine adrenal cortex cells in vitro. Horm Metab Res 13:95-98

Eggens U, Bahr V, Oelkers W (1987) Effects of β-lipotropin, β-endorphin, γ2-melanotropin and corticotropin on steroid production by isolated human adrenocortical cells. J Clin Chem Clin Biochem 25:779-783

Eipper BA, Mains RE (1980) Structure and biosynthesis of proadrenocorticotropin/endorphin and related peptides. Endocr Rev 1:1-27

Giagnoni G, Sabol SL, Nirenberg M (1977) Synthesis of opiate peptides by a clonal pituitary tumor cell line. Proc Natl Acad Sci USA 74:2259-2263

Gibson A, Ginsburg M, Hall M, Hart SL (1979) The effects of opioid drugs and of lithium on steroidogenesis in rat adrenal cell suspensions. Br J Pharmacol 65:671-676

Goverde HJM, Pesman GJ, Smals AGH (1988) The melanotropin potentiating factor and β-endorphin do not modulate the γ2-melanotropin or adrenocorticotropin-induced corticosteroidogenesis in purified isolated rat adrenal cells. Neuropeptides 12:125-130

Guaza C, Zubiaur M, Borrell J (1986) Corticosteroido genesis modulation by β-endorphin and dynorphin1-17 in isolated rat adrenocortical cells. Peptides 7:237-240

Guillemin R, Vargo T, Rossier J, Minich S, Ling N, Rivier C, Vale W, Bloom F (1977) β-endorphin and adrenocorticotropin are secreted concomitantly by the pituitary gland. Science 197:1367- 1369

Güllner H-G, Gill JR (1983) Beta endorphin selectively stimulates aldosterone secretion in hypophysectomized, nephrectomized dogs. J Clin Invest 71:124-128

Kem DC, Feldman M, Starkweather G, Li CH (1985) Effect of human β-endorphin on plasma aldosterone concentrations in normal human subjects. J Clin Endocrinol Metab 60:440-443

Lamberts SWJ, Bons EG, del Pozo E (1983) The met-enkephalin analog FK-824 and naloxone do not directly influence cortisol secretion by cultured human adrenocortical cells. Life Sci 32:755-758

Mains R, Eipper E, Ling N (1977) Common precursor to corticotropins and endorphins. Proc Natl Acad Sci USA 74:3014-3018

Matsuoka H, Mulrow PJ, LI CH (1980) β-Lipotropin: a new aldosterone-stimulating factor. Science 209:307-308

Matsuoka H, Mulrow PJ, Franco-Saez R (1981) Effects of β- lipotropin and β-lipotropin-derived peptides on aldosterone production in the rat adrenal gland. J Clin Invest 68:752-759

Nakao K, Nakai Y, Oki S, Horii K, Imura H (1978) Presence of immunoreactive β-endorphin in normal human plasma. J Clin Invest 62:1395-1398

Nakao K, Nakai Y, Jingami H, Oki S, Fukata J, Imura H (1979) Substantial rise of plasma β-endorphin levels after insulin- induced hypoglycemia in human subjects. J Clin Endocrinol Metab 49:838-841

Pham-Huu-Trung MT, Smitter ND, Bogyo A, Bertagna X, Girard F (1982) Responses of isolated guinea-pig adrenal cells to ACTH and pro-opiocortin-derived peptides. Endocrinology 110:1819-1821

Pham-Huu-Trung M-T, Bogyo A, Smitter ND, Girard F (1985) Effects of proopiomelanocortin peptides and angiotensin II on steroidogenesis in isolated aldosteronoma cells. J Clin Endocrinol Metab 61:467-471

Rabinowe SL, Taylor T, Dluhy RG, Williams GH (1985) β- Endorphin stimulates plasma renin and aldosterone release in normal human subjects. J Clin Endocrinol Metab 60:485-489

Rácz K, Gláz E, Kiss R, Lada GY, Varga I, Vida S, di Gleria K, Medzihradszky K, Lichtwald K, Vecsei P (1980) Adrenal cortex — a newly recognized peripheral site of action of enkephalins. Biochem Biophys Res Commun 97:1346-1353

Shanker G, Sharma RK (1979) β-Endorphin stimulates corticosterone synthesis in isolated rat adrenal cells. Biochem Biophys Res Commun 86:1-5

Simantov R, Snyder SH (1977) Opiate receptor binding in the pituitary gland. Brain Res 124:178-184

Szalay KSZ (1981) Effect of pituitary intermediate lobe extract on steroid production by the isolated zona glomerulosa and fasciculata cells. Acta Physiol Acad Sci Hung 57:225-231

Szalay KSZ, Stark E (1981) Effect of beta-endorphin on the steroid production of isolated zona glomerulosa and zona fasciculata cells. Life Sci 29:1355-1361

Taylor T, Dluhy RG, Williams GD (1983) β-Endorphin suppresses adrenocorticotropin and cortisol levels in normal human subjects. J Clin Endocrinol Metab 57:592-596

Vale W, Rivier C, Yang L, Minich, Guillemin R (1978) Effects of purified hypothalamic corticotropin-releasing factor and other substances on the secretion of adrenocorticotropin and β-endorphin-like immunoactivities in vitro. Endocrinology 103:1910-1915

Washburn DD, Kem DC, Orth DN, Nicholson WE, Chretien M, Mount CD (1982) Effect of β-lipotropin on aldosterone production in the isolated rat adrenal cell preparation. J Clin Endocrinol Metab 54:613-618

Wiedemann E, Saito T, Linfoot JA, Li CH (1979) Specific radioimmunoassay of human β-endorphin in unextracted plasma. J Clin Endocrinol Metab 49:478-480

Effects of Blood-Borne Endorphin and Other POMC-Derived Peptides on Brain Functions in Man[*]

J. BORN and H.L. FEHM

Introduction

Hormones of the hypothalamus-pituitary adrenal (HPA) axis are released into the blood as part of the organism's response to stressful stimuli. These hormones do not only act on peripheral tissues but feed back to the central nervous system, thus forming part of an afferent humoral system modulating a great variety of brain functions, including functions not directly related to the endocrine regulation such as sensory processing and sleep (Fig. 1). In rats, the systemic administration of the proopiomelanocortin (POMC) peptides ACTH 4-10 and

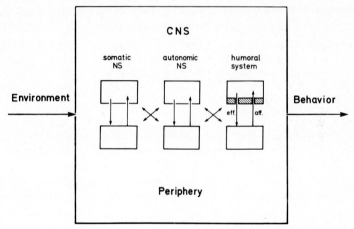

Fig. 1. Concept of the regulation of behavioral adaptation. Behavioral adaptation relies on an intense communication between the central nervous system (CNS) and the periphery. Three systems, each comprising an efferent and afferent branch, are responsible for the flow of information: the somatic and autonomic nervous systems and the humoral system, the latter transferring information at a slower rate. According to this concept, hormones released upon stress from the pituitary do not only act on peripheral tissue but feed back to the brain modulating various central nervous functions

---
[*] This work was supported by a grant from the Deutsche Forschungsgemeinschaft (to H.L.F.). The study was approved by the committee on Research Involving Human Subjects of the University of Ulm.

β-endorphin has been shown to delay extinction of conditioned avoidance behavior and to affect the hippocampal θ rhythm (de Wied and Jolles 1982; de Wied et al. 1978; Urban and de Wied 1976). Receptors located at the blood–brain barrier and in the circumventricular organs are possible mediators of the central effects of these hormones after peripheral administration (see, e.g., Meisenberg and Simmons 1983; van Houten and Posner 1983).

The present experiments on afferent influences of β-endorphin belonged to a series of studies which aimed at demonstrating influences of HPA hormones on nonendocrine central nervous functions in humans (Born et al. 1990,1989a). Scalp-recorded auditory event-related brain potentials (ERPs) reflecting stages of sensory processing were taken as a bioassay which in previous experiments has been proved to be sensitive to influences of peptides after systemic administration (Born et al. 1987a,b). The very early components of the auditory ERP (latency < 10 ms; BAEPs) reflect neuronal transmission within the auditory nerve and in brain stem nuclei of the auditory pathways. The late components of the ERP (latency > 100 ms) are associated with the cortical processing of the stimulus and reflect different aspects of attention.

In the present experiments, changes in BAEPs and in late attention-related ERP components were assessed following intravenous administration of two different doses of β-endorphin in healthy human subjects. In view of similar actions of ACTH and β-endorphin on certain types of behavior in rats, it has been speculated that the central actions of these POMC peptides are mediated in part by the same receptor system (de Wied and Jolles 1982; Jacquet 1979). Therefore, the pattern of changes in ERPs following β-endorphin were compared with the effects obtained following administration of ACTH-related petides in two previous studies (Born et al. 1987b; Born 1989).

Method

Twelve male adults (of normal hearing, nonsmoking, aged between 20 and 33 years) voluntarily participated in the experiments. At least 12 h prior to experimental sessions they had to abstain from coffee and alcoholic beverages. Sessions were scheduled for 2.00 or 3.00 p.m. and lasted for 2 h. One hour before experimental testing, subjects intravenously received either placebo (saline solution) or 0.1 or 1.0 mg β-endorphin, according to a double-blind latin square design. Substances were infused over a period of about 10 min. Any two of the three experimental sessions of each subject were at least 10 days apart.

In each session, BAEPs and attention-related ERP components were recorded with the order of recordings balanced across subjects. BAEPs were obtained to series of rarefaction clicks presented at three different intensities (80, 60, 40 dB HL) and with two different stimulus rates (39, 10 clicks/s) resulting in a total of six conditions. BAEP recordings and analysis were performed according to standards described previously (Born et al. 1989b).

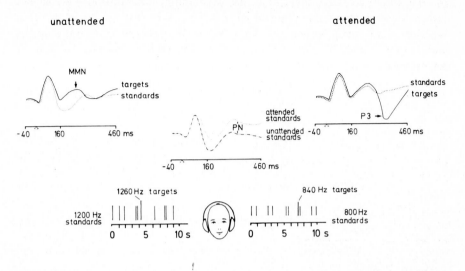

Fig. 2. Selective attention task. *Bottom:* Subjects were presented with sequences of tone pips concurrently presented to the right and left ear. Sequences in each ear consisted of frequent standard and rare target pips. The subjects were to count target pips in one ear at a time, ignoring all pips in the opposite ear. *Upper panels:* During attention performance, ERPs to the different types of tone pips (attended and unattended standards; attended and unattended targets) were recorded (vertex negative is upward). From these ERPs the following components were extracted: (1, *middle*) PN (a measure of selective attention), a negative potential shift in ERPs to attended standards as compared to the ERPs to unattended standard; (2, *right*) P3, a positive potential shift about 300 ms post stimulus in ERPs to attended target pips compared to the ERPs to attended standard pips; (P3 reflects short term memory updating subsequent to the identification of a task-relevant target); (3, *left*) MMN, a negative potential deflection in ERPs to unattended targets compared to the ERPs to unattended standards. MMN is a sign of the brain's automatic processing of stimulus deviance

ERP indicators of attention were measured in a dichotic listening paradigm (Hillyard et al. 1973; Fig. 2). Recording techniques were the same as in previous studies (e.g., Born et al. 1989a) and will not be described in detail. The dichotic listening paradigm consisted of sequences of tone pips (60 ms, 60 dB SPL) delivered through earphones to the subject's left and right ear (interstimulus intervals: 250-1250 ms). Tone pips were presented randomly at four different frequencies: frequent standard pips for the different ears were 800 and 1200 Hz; rare target tones (10% probable) were of slightly higher pitch than the standard tones, i.e., 840 and 1260 Hz. In four blocks, each containing about 400 pips, subjects had to silently count the targets in one ear, and simultaneously to ignore all pips in the opposite ear. The ear to be attended to was counter-balanced across blocks. Earphones were reversed after half of the blocks, and half of the subjects started the experiment with reversed earphones. Between any two blocks a short break was used to check for the subject's count. To avoid eye movement artifacts, subjects were instructed to fix their gaze on a centrally located dot during attention performance.

ERPs were averaged separately for the different tone pips and recording sites used in this study (Fz, Cz, Pz, referenced to linked earlobe electrodes). Measurements derived from the ERPs to the different tone pips were:

1. Processing negativity (PN), indexing selectivity of attention. PN was determined as the mean amplitude difference between ERPs to attended and unattended standard tones within 0-460 ms post stimulus.
2. *P3* in ERPs to attended target pips P3 amplitude was defined as the mean amplitude difference between ERPs to the attended targets and ERPs to the attended standards within 280-600 ms post stimulus. P3 latency was determined with reference to the maximum positive amplitude within the same latency bin.
3. Mismatch negativity (MMN), reflecting the automatic processing of stimulus deviance (Näätänen et al. 1980), was determined as the mean amplitude difference between ERPs to unattended target and unattended standard pips, within 180-360 ms post stimulus.

Immediately before and after the ERP recordings, blood pressure, heart rate, and oral temperature were measured, and blood samples were collected to determine plasma cortisol and ACTH concentrations. Statistical analysis was, in general, based on analysis of variance (ANOVA).

Results

PN and MMN dominated in recordings from anterior recording sites (Fz, Cz) in all treatment conditions; P3 amplitude was largest in recordings from Pz (ANOVA main effects for site of electrode $p < 0.01$). The infusion of β-endorphin reduced PN, with this effect being stronger after low (0.1 mg, $p < 0.05$) than after high (1.0 mg, n.s.) doses (Fig. 3). P3 amplitude was also reduced following administration of 0.1 mg β-endorphin by more than 30% ($p < 0.05$), whereas the administration of 1.0 mg β-endorphin was ineffective. None of the peptide treatments had a systematic effect on P3 latency or MMN.

There were no consistent influences of β-endorphin on latencies or amplitudes of BAEPs (Table 1). As is indicated in Table 2, neither cardiovascular parameters nor temperature were systematically influenced by β-endorphin. There was a slight increase in plasma cortisol and ACTH concentrations following both low and high doses of β-endorphin, but these changes failed to reach the 5% level of statistical significance.

The average deviations of the target counts from the correct value (a rough behavioral measure of attention performance) were (mean ± SEM) 1.9 ± 0.3 following placebo, 2.1 ± 0.7 following 0.1 mg β-endorphin, and 2.0 ± 0.5 following 1.0 mg. These values did not differ significantly from each other.

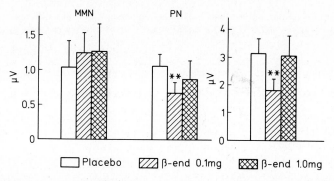

Fig. 3. MMN, PN (both averaged across recordings from Fz and Cz), and P3 amplitude (at Pz), for the three treatment conditions (placebo, 0.1, and 1.0 mg β-endorphin, i.v.). ** $p < 0.05$ for a pairwise comparison with results from the placebo session

Table 1. Mean (± SEM) latencies of BAEP wave III and V, which could be most reliably identified, for the different treatment and stimulus conditions[a]

		Placebo	β–End (0.1 mg)	β–End (1.0 mg)
Wave III	80 dBHL	3.82 (0.14)	3.79 (0.11)	3.78 (0.12)
	60 dBHL	4.06 (0.08)	4.08 (0.07)	3.97 (0.07)
	40 dBHL	4.83 (0.11)	4.85 (0.09)	4.94 (0.09)
Wave V	80 dBHL	5.73 (0.07)	5.80 (0.06)*	5.77 (0.06)
	60 dBHL	6.21 (0.10)	6.21 (0.09)	6.14 (0.08)
	40 dBHL	6.99 (0.12)	7.03 (0.11)	6.92 (0.10)
Wave III	10 clicks/s	4.22 (0.11)	4.22 (0.09)	4.13 (0.06)
	39 clicks/s	4.29 (0.08)	4.28 (0.08)	4.33 (0.11)
Wave V	10 clicks/s	6.21 (0.09)	6.21 (0.08)	6.19 (0.07)
	39 clicks/s	6.45 (0.09)	6.48 (0.08)	6.37 (0.09)

[a]Latencies for a given intensity condition represent averages across both stimulus rate conditions and vice versa.
** $p < 0.05$, * $p < 0.10$ in comparisons with the placebo condition.

Table 2. Cardiovascular parameters and body temperature for the different treatment conditions[a]

	Placebo	β-End (0.1 mg)	β-End (1.0 mg)
Cortisol (μg/dl)	6.7 (0.5)	8.2 (1.9)	7.3 (0.9)
ACTH (pg/ml)	47.6 (12.7)	85.1 (15.4)*	79.7 (17.1)
Oral temperature (C°)	36.6 (0.07)	36.5 (0.07)	36.7 (0.07)
Heart Rate (b/min)	67.1 (2.8)	67.5 (2.5)	64.7 (2.7)
Blood pressure (mmHg)			
Systolic	114.0 (2.0)	112.4 (1.8)	111.2 (2.5)
Diastolic	63.0 (2.5)	63.1 (1.9)	62.4 (2.6)

[a]Values represent averages across measures taken before and after ERP recordings. ** $p <$ 0.05, * $p < 0.10$ in pairwise comparisons with the placebo condition.

Neither were there any systematic differences among the treatment conditions with respect to feelings of concentration, activation, and tiredness as rated on seven-point rating scales at the end of the sessions. At this time subjects were not able to identify correctly the treatment they had received.

Discussion

Results from the present study demonstrate afferent humoral influences of β-endorphin on stimulus-evoked brain potentials after systemic administration in humans. While BAEPs were not affected, PN and P3 amplitude were significantly reduced following administration of 0.1 mg β-endorphin. Changes in the same direction following 1.0 mg β-endorphin were smaller and non-significant. The pattern of actions suggests an impairing influence of low doses of β-endorphin on electrophysiological correlates of selective attention in humans.

The central nervous effects of β-endorphin cannot be reduced to changes in heart rate, blood pressure, or oral temperature, for these parameters remained unchanged. Fluctuations in hormonal concentrations (plasma ACTH and cortisol) during the β-endorphin conditions also appeared to be marginal and probably cannot account for the central effects of β-endorphin.

However, a previous study has shown that strong increases in plasma ACTH (300 pg/ml) induce ERP changes resembling those of β-endorphin (Born 1989). The main results of that study, comparing effects of ACTH 1-39 (infused i.v. at a constant rate of 2 U/h, from 1 h prior to the recordings until the end of the experiment) and placebo on ERPs in 13 healthy male students are summarized in Tables 3 and 4. Like β-endorphin, ACTH did not consistently influence BAEPs or MMN; ACTH also reduced PN and significantly decreased P3 amplitude. Moreover, we have been able to show that the 4-10 fragment of ACTH is sufficient for inducing significant reductions in PN (Born et al. 1987b):

Table 3. Mean (± SEM) amplitudes of PN, P3, and MMN in recordings from midline electrode locations (Fz, Cz, Pz; references against linked earlobe electrodes): placebo vs.ACTH 1- 39

	Fz	Cz	Pz
PN (µV)			
Placebo	1.14 (0.15)	1.05 (0.16)	0.39 (0.17)
ACTH	0.84 (0.17)**	0.82 (0.20)**	0.36 (0.11)
P3 (µV)			
Placebo	0.01 (0.97)	1.83 (0.97)	2.54 (0.59)
ACTH	0.03 (0.77)	1.19 (0.79)	1.63 (0.62)**
MMN (µV)			
Placebo	1.37 (0.34)	0.82 (0.27)	0.18 (0.26)
ACTH	1.37 (0.23)	0.82 (0.28)	0.48 (0.26)

** $p < 0.05$ in one-tailed comparisons with the placebo condition

Table 4. Plasma cortisol and ACTH concentrations collapsed across values obtained immediately before and after ERP recordings

	Cortisol (µg/dl)	ACTH (pg/ml)
Placebo	7.7 (0.8)	47.4 (12.8)
ACTH	24.3 (2.0)**	641.1 (105.2)**

** $p < 0.05$ in comparisons with the placebo condition.

In that study with logarithmically increasing doses of ACTH 4-10 (0.1 mg, 1.0 mg, 10 mg, vs. placebo) the decrease in PN linearly increased in magnitude.

In sum, the present study together with results from previous experiments indicate that the POMC peptides β-endorphin and ACTH impair ERP indicators of selective attention in humans. Other ERP components, such as MMN or brain stem potentials, were not affected by the peptides. The findings are consistent with the hypothesis that central actions of ACTH and β-endorphin (after systemic administration) are mediated through the same receptor system in man. It is remarkable, however, that effects of β-endorphin were confined to the lower doses of 0.1 mg, but did not reach significance with the higher doses of 1.0 mg. Effects of ACTH 4-10, by contrast, linearly increased in strength up to doses of 10 mg. Thus, further studies need to clarify whether and to what extent the dynamics of influences on selective attention in humans is different for these two types of POMC derivatives.

Acknowledgement. The authors would like to thank Mrs. A. Otterbein and Mr. E. Seidel for technical assistance.

References

Born J (1989) Untersuchungen zur afferenten humoralen Beeinflussung zentralnervöser Aktivität beim Menschen. Habilitationsschrift, University of Ulm

Born J, Bathelt B, Pietrowsky R, Pauschinger P, Fehm HL (1990) Influences of peripheral adrenocorticotropin 1-39 (ACTH) and human corticotropin releasing hormone (h-CRH) on human auditory evoked potentials (AEP). Psychopharmacology (Berlin) 101: 34-38

Born J, Bothor R, Pietrowsky R, Fehm-Wolfsdorf G, Pauschinger P, Fehm HL (1987a) Influences of vasopressin and oxytocin on human event-related brain potentials in an attention task. J Psychophysiol 4:351-360

Born J, Bräuninger W, Fehm-Wolfsdorf G, Voigt KH, Pauschinger P, Fehm HL (1987b) Dose-dependent influences on electrophysiological signs of attention in humans after neuropeptide ACTH 4-10. Exp Brain Res 67:85-92

Born J, Kern W, Pietrowsky R, Sittig W, Fehm HL (1989a) Fragments of ACTH affect electrophysiological signs of controlled stimulus processing in humans. Psychopharmacology (Berlin) 99: 439-444

Born J, Späth-Schwalbe E, Pietrowsky R, Porzsolt F, Fehm HL (1989b) Neurophysiological effects of recombinant interferon gamma and alpha in man. Clin Physiol Biochem 7:119-127

De Wied D, Bohus B, van Ree JM, Urban I (1978) Behavioral and electrophysiological effects of peptides related to lipotropin (β-LPH). J Pharmacol Exp Ther 204:570-580

De Wied D, Jolles J (1982) Neuropeptides derived from proopiocortin: behavioral, physiological, and neurochemical effects. Physiol Rev 62:976-1059

Hillyard SA, Hink RF, Schwent VL, Picton TW (1973) Electrical signs of selective attention in the human brain. Science 182:177- 180

Jacquet YF (1979) Dual mechanisms mediating opiate effects? Science 205:425-426

Meisenberg G, Simmons WH (1983) Peptides and the blood–brain barrier. Life Sci 32:2611-2623

Näätänen R, Gaillard AWK, Mantysalo S (1980) Brain potentials of voluntary and involuntary attention. In: Kornhuber HH, Deecke L (ed) Motivation, motor and sensory processes of the brain: electrical potentials, behaviour and clinical use. Elsevier, Amsterdam, pp 343-348

Van Houten M, Posner BI (1983) Circumventricular organs: receptors and mediators of direct peptide hormone action on brain. Adv Metab Disord 10:269-289

Urban I, de Wied D (1976) Changes in excitability of the theta activity generating substrate by ACTH 4-10 in the rat. Exp Brain Res 24:325-344